D1442126

Louis-Guy D

EVERYTHING YOU NEED TO KNOW

TO HAVE GREAT-

LOOKING

hair

Louis-Guy D

EVERYTHING YOU NEED TO KNOW TO HAVE GREAT-LOOKING

hair

by Louis Gignac

with Jacqueline Warsaw

Designed by Susan Niles

PHOTOGRAPHY: GEORGE BARKENTIN
ILLUSTRATIONS: CARMEN VARRICCHIO

● THE VIKING PRESS ● NEW YORK ●

A Note on Products

Throughout this book great care has been taken to name specific commercial and salon products and treatments for hair care, but manufacturers often discontinue products and some listed here may no longer be available.

Printed in the United States of America
9 8 7 6 5 4

Photograph on page 132 by Nobu, courtesy *Vogue*.
Copyright © 1980 by The Condé Nast Publications, Inc.

To my mother

Very special thanks to:
 Jeannine Gignac, my wife
 Jean Michel, my son
 Carole Shapiro, who was with me when
  the idea was born
 Geraldine Taaffe, who nurtured and
  guided this effort from its beginning,
  four years ago

My deep appreciation to:
 Edith Raymond Locke, who made me
 Andrea Quinn Robinson, who believed in me
 Joanna Brown, who steered me to the
  right coauthor

And to those in my life who encouraged
  and supported me throughout my career:
 Nonnie Eilers Moore
 Mary Simons
 Esther Block
 Nancy Evans
 Rollene Saal
 Mallen De Santis
 Sandy Horvitz
 Peggy Moore
 Patricia Orlando
 Jim Kaufman, my lawyer
 Guy Hoffman and Gregory Schaedle, my
  partners
 And to all my clients

Sincere thanks to the team that made this
  book possible:
 Jacqueline Warsaw, who wrote it the way
  I couldn't
 Meredith Bernstein, my agent
 Amanda Vaill, my editor
 Elizabeth Dranow Gutner, Coordinator
 George Barkentin, for his fine photography
 Susan Niles, for her design and art direction

My staff at Louis-Guy D:
 Constance Hartnett, Coloring Director
 Elsa Serra, Makeup & Color Coordinator
 Corinne Lozach, Stylist
 Peter Raymond Mikell, Stylist
 Rafael Damiano, Stylist

PREFACE

I can give you the best cut in the world, but if your hair isn't healthy, it will never look great.

That's the difference between this book and others—most of them are filled with trivia and gossip that have nothing to do with you and your hair's well-being. But this book is the culmination of twenty years of coiffuring everyone, from the Manhattan élite to the college student, and it's devoted solely to giving you the basics: a healthy head of naturally beautiful hair.

I've done hair seminars and makeovers on university campuses from coast to coast. My tips and advice are on the pages of all the great fashion and beauty magazines worldwide: *Vogue, Harper's Bazaar, Glamour, Mademoiselle, Seventeen* . . . over fifty different magazines in all. Their editors, those amazing women who travel to the ends of the earth in their quest for newness and beauty, are my clients. They have been creating with me for two decades. But—whether they're university students or beauty editors—I've always encouraged and taught my clients how to "do it themselves," to follow regimens based on solid knowledge and common sense. There are honestly no tricks or gimmicks in having healthy, shining hair.

It's just a matter of knowing what you have and how to make it fabulous. So if you would like to know simply how to have absolutely great-looking hair, read on. You're the reason I wrote this book.

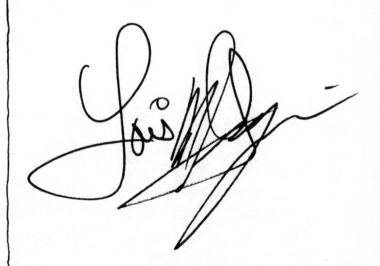

ACKNOWLEDGMENTS

My sincere thanks to the editors of the following publications who have shared the "Louis-Guy D Way" with their readers:

American Baby
American Home
Bride's
Co-ed
Cosmopolitan
Daily News
Denver Post
Eye
Family Circle
Glamour
Good Housekeeping
Harper's Bazaar
Houston Chronicle
Ladies' Home Journal
L'Officiel
Mademoiselle
New York
Redbook
Seventeen
Shop
Talk
Teen
The New York Times
Time
Town & Country
Viva
Vogue
Vogue (Great Britain)
Vogue (France)
Vogue (Italy)
Votre Beauté (American and French editions)
W.
W.W.
Weight Watchers
Woman's Day
Women's Wear Daily
Working Woman

My appreciation for their participation:

Clairol
L'Oréal
Revlon
Boyd's of Madison Avenue
Riviera, Inc.

Special thanks to:
Dr. Richard C. Gibbs, Clinical Professor of Dermatology at New York University School of Medicine
Dr. Richard S. Rivlin, Professor of Medicine at Cornell University Medical College and Chief of Nutrition at New York Hospital-Cornell Medical Center and Memorial Sloan-Kettering Cancer Center
Dr. Judy Stern, Sc.D., Associate Professor of Nutrition at University of California, Davis Campus
Dr. John F. Corbett, Clairol
Verne Silverman, Clairol
Dr. John Penicnak, L'Oréal
Dr. Gus Klein, Revlon

C O N T E N T S

Louis-Guy D
EVERYTHING YOU NEED TO KNOW
TO HAVE GREAT-
LOOKING
hair

The Louis-Guy D way

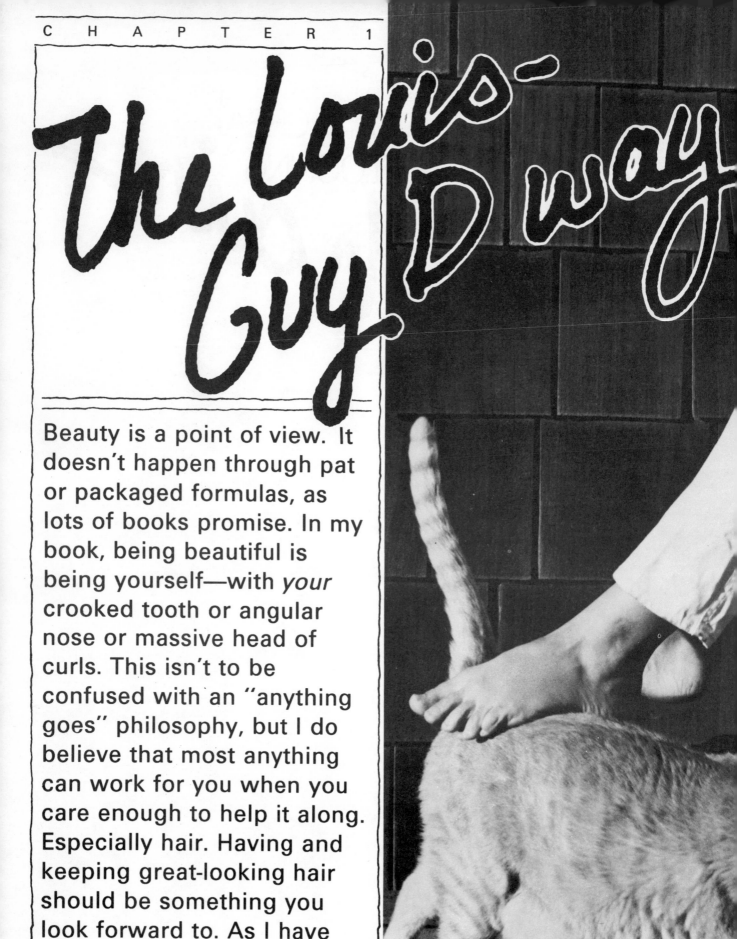

Beauty is a point of view. It doesn't happen through pat or packaged formulas, as lots of books promise. In my book, being beautiful is being yourself—with *your* crooked tooth or angular nose or massive head of curls. This isn't to be confused with an "anything goes" philosophy, but I do believe that most anything can work for you when you care enough to help it along. Especially hair. Having and keeping great-looking hair should be something you look forward to. As I have and still do.

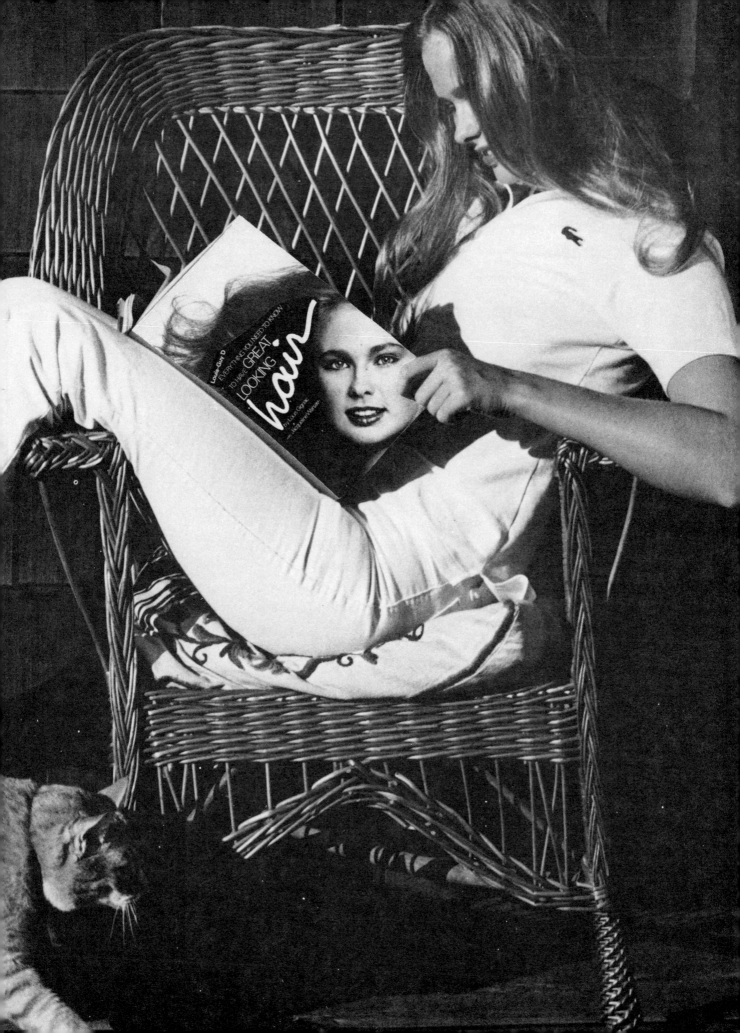

Putting one's philosophy down on paper seems inappropriate when putting it into action is what beliefs are all about. But in order to acquaint you with what's to come in my book, I think it's only fair to share with you some of the concepts on which the "Louis-Guy D way" is built. The easiest way for me to explain these concepts is to spotlight key words and phrases that briefly express what I mean:

Simple—
hair that's uncomplicated, uncluttered, and un-done-up.
Classic—
hair that's never out of style,
never old-fashioned.
Natural—
hair that's swinging and bouncy, not plastered
or pinned down.
Healthy—
hair that's clean, shiny, and well nourished.
Liberated—
hair that's fresh, full of its own motion
and unhampered by teasing,
spraying, faking.
Carefree—
hair that's easy to manage by yourself, free from time-consuming daily
rituals and weekly visits to the beauty salon.
Individual—
hair that best expresses who *you* are, not someone else.

This is not a book of rules, nor is it intended to preach. Certainly, it is full of what I prefer people to have and do, but I'm also a firm believer in "doing your own thing." So if you're looking for dogma here, you won't find it. But if you're looking for encouragement and the courage to make a change and be free, you'll not be disappointed. The Louis-Guy D way is philosophy in action. It's a way of being and living and enjoying. It's what excites me most about every beautiful head of hair I meet.

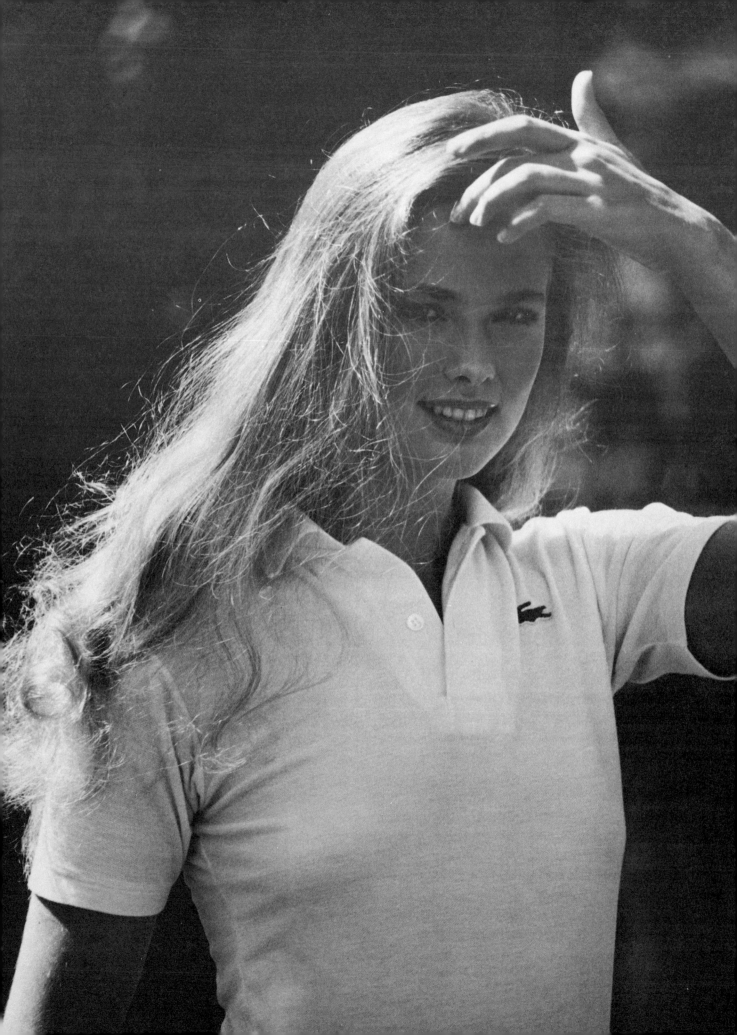

Facts & Fables

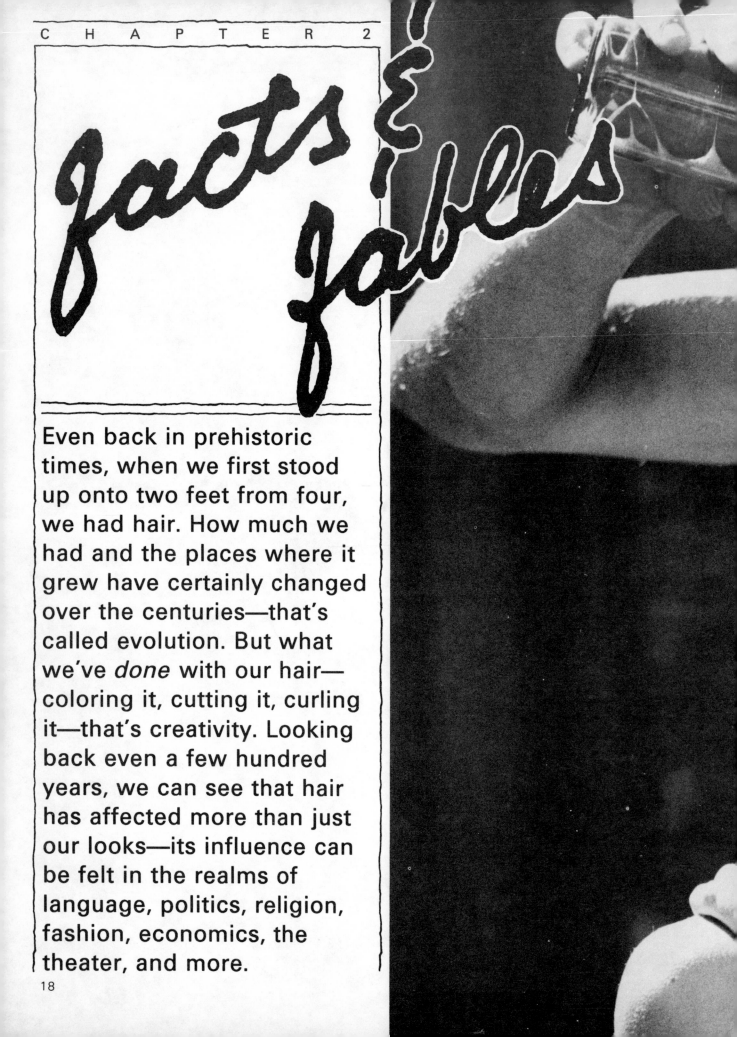

Even back in prehistoric times, when we first stood up onto two feet from four, we had hair. How much we had and the places where it grew have certainly changed over the centuries—that's called evolution. But what we've *done* with our hair—coloring it, cutting it, curling it—that's creativity. Looking back even a few hundred years, we can see that hair has affected more than just our looks—its influence can be felt in the realms of language, politics, religion, fashion, economics, the theater, and more.

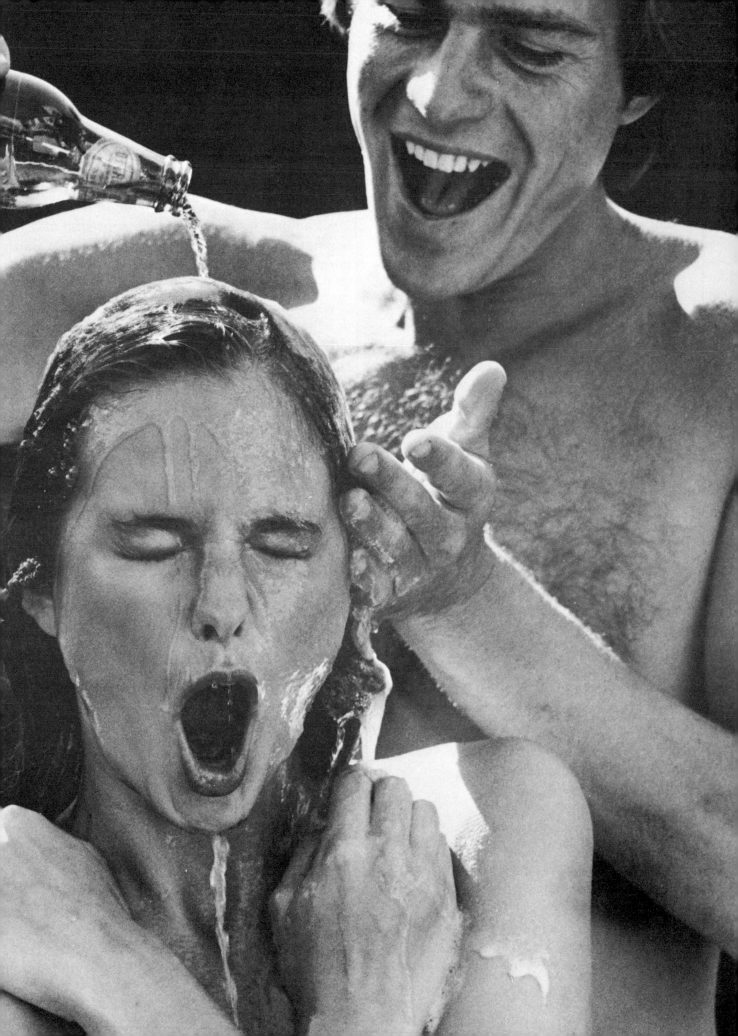

These are marvelous words—some slang, others more serious, but all wonderfully funny and visually rich—to describe different kinds of hair and different degrees of hairiness:

Blizzard head— slang for blonde.
Beaver—slang term for a film extra with a full natural beard.
Bob—hairstyle introduced by actress Irene Castle in 1914.
Brick top—slang for an auburn-haired person.
Cookie Duster—a mustache.
Face Lace—a beard.
Fly Rink—a bald head.
Hitchhike—a finger wave.

Flames—a wig or toupee.
Mouse tail—a pencil-thin mustache.

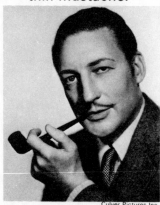

Culver Pictures Inc.

And while we're on mustaches, someone once said that "a kiss without a mustache is like an egg without salt."

All this talk about hair simply confirms the part it has played in history. Sometimes its role was purely practical: In the sixteenth and seventeenth centuries, tennis balls were handstuffed with human hair to give them bounce (how's that for sensible recycling?). But sometimes it was inspirational: In the early nineteenth century, Lord Byron's long locks so inspired all the young romantics of his day that they were copied—causing the first "natural look." Fashion has always influenced the way we wear our hair or wigs. Did you

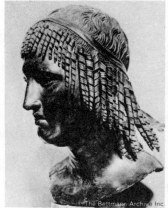

The Bettmann Archive Inc.

know, for example, many Roman portrait busts were made with adjustable wigs so they could be kept up-to-date? And that in England, when Charles II led fashionable men into wearing black wigs, the demand for black hair for the wig-making process became so obsessive that children often had their hair cut off while walking in the streets?

Gray hair, on the other hand, seems to have been *out* of fashion for the ancient Egyptians. In fact, they had a prescription to prevent it, which consisted of 1 part paw of dog, 1 part kernel of date, and 1 part hoof of donkey. These ingredients were to be cooked in an earthenware pot and later used to anoint the head.

Color through the Ages. Hair color—gray or otherwise—has stirred up some mad fantasies through the centuries. Way back in ancient Rome, a yellow wig was obligatory for prostitutes, who were licensed and taxed—don't ask why, but yellow hair became the rage for society ladies. And as for Rome's famous fiddler, Nero, he used gold dust for powdering his hair. Pink, gray, blue, and white were also popular. In sixteenth-century England, Queen Elizabeth I started a new fad: Many women dyed their hair red as a gesture of loyalty to her. Then Henri IV set a fashion when he used dark powder to hide his gray hair.

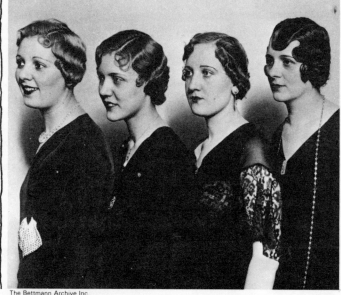

The Bettmann Archive Inc.

But real color fantasies seem to have started more recently: In 1916 the French hairdresser Antoine invented colored wigs for his clients in strange and bright colors—orange, blue, purple, red, snow white—*any* color, in fact, that had no relation to real hair.

Now let's dip into blondes. Did you know that Aphrodite was a blonde? And that Poppaea dyed her hair blonde at Nero's request? Blonde seemed to be aspired to as well as an inspiration. The famous Venetian artists Titian, Palma Vecchio, and Botticelli painted blonde hair, even though blonde hair was an exception in Italy.

Hair Mythology. Biologists call hair a "secondary sexual characteristic," and the mythology that has sprung up around it bears out the label. Not for nothing did the church fathers insist that women cover their heads to keep men from temptation! Rituals and customs throughout history seem to keep hair and sexuality—or hair and love—interestingly wedded. For example, early Irish custom was for the wife to give her husband two bracelets made from her own hair; and the locket with a strand of hair inside is still with us. From Lady Godiva to Rapunzel, long hair has always been full of

symbolism. (*Length* shouldn't be confused with an *abundance* of hair, which was sometimes supposed to indicate wantoness in women—and sexual energy in men.) Here are a few facts: From the fourteenth to the seventeenth century, it was customary for brides to wear their long hair hanging down, spilling over their shoulders as a recognized symbol of virginity. Certainly short, curly hair would

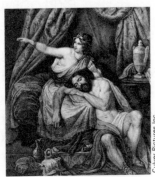

not have been a big draw in those days.

Ancients saw hair as a source of strength and power, and refrained from cutting it lest it damage those assets. The classic myth of depriving a man of his strength by cutting his hair is perfectly illustrated by the story of Samson's shorn locks.

And then in the twelfth

century the church protested against the vanity of men who wore long hair, and bishops were permitted to carry scissors with them to lop off locks.

Priests of Bonism, a pre-Buddhist religion still found in Tibet, sometimes have hair a dozen feet in length coiled atop their heads like a snake, a symbol of immortality.

But it's in Hollywood, land of magic and make-believe, that the Lady Godivas and the Samsons of today have made their mark: Wigs were designed for Jeannette MacDonald to widen her face and help shorten her long neck. In 1938, Jeannette wore a bright red wig in the film *Sweethearts* because the film was changed at the last minute from black and white to color. Veronica Lake was transformed

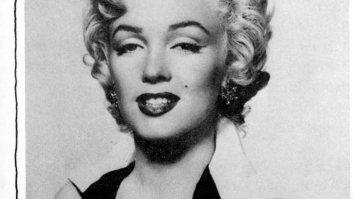

Culver Pictures Inc.

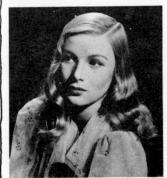

Culver Pictures Inc.

from pigtailed girl-next-door to siren by a Paramount hairdresser. (Although Lake had a good bosom, anti-cleavage legislation prohibited costumers from using it, so the hair carried the look instead.) Then there was Mary Pickford, with her fa-

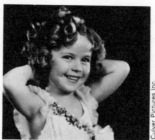
Culver Pictures Inc.

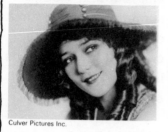
Culver Pictures Inc.

mous curls (the inspiration, later, for Shirley Temple's curls). When Perce Westmore cut bangs for Bette Davis it started a rage for the style. The "wash-tub" hairdo of Hepburn's also sent women off trying to copy it.

Other Hollywood innovators made Rita Hayworth a strawberry blonde at the request of Jack Warner for her role in *Strawberry Blonde*. She had started her career in Hollywood as Marguerite Cansino, a black-haired beauty who Harry Cohn hoped would rival Hedy Lamarr. She received rave reviews for the *Blonde* part, changed her personality considerably, divorced her

first husband, and married Orson Welles. Just goes to show you what blonde hair can do.

Why did I delve back into time to unearth some of the funnier follies and fantasies we attached to hair? Because so many of today's myths are simply new versions of the same old themes. I find it curious that other parts of the body escape myth-making. But not hair.

EXPLODING THE MYTHS

Hair mythology doesn't just live in history books, though; there are hundreds of old wives' tales that have a curious way of hanging on forever and being accepted as fact—even by the women who are my clients! Just when you think you've laid one to rest, it resurfaces, slightly altered, but bearing an obvious resemblance to its former self.

I was surprised to find my "myth list" mushrooming as I asked client after client to recall a pet myth about hair tucked away somewhere in her

memory. Amazingly, more than one myth per person usually turned up. A few were so far-out that I could only attribute their creation to some local witch doctor. Others were highly imaginative. The full moon played a powerful role in many. The following list of myths—each with a corresponding column of facts to set them right—highlights the fictions most commonly believed and quoted. But I'm sure that as quickly as these are corrected, others will spring up to take their place. After all, what is life without the spice of a few creative myths?

Myth:	**Fact:**
Beer is a good rinse and setting lotion.	Beer will not give your hair more body or shine. Just the opposite, in fact. It will dull your hair, dry out the scalp, and eventually create a dandruff problem. My advice is to drink the beer instead; it's a more effective way to "glow," but remember, it's fattening, too.
Myth:	**Fact:**
The less you shampoo your hair, the healthier it will get.	It'll get unhealthy because it'll get dirty! Also, oily hair isn't pretty.

Myth:
When a woman is menstruating, she should avoid having her hair permanent waved, colored, or blow-dried.

Fact:
Chemical processes have nothing to do with your monthly cycle. The structure of your hair is not related to your body's reproductive structure.

Myth:
The more frequently you cut your hair, the faster it will grow.

Fact:
Cutting by itself does not affect the growth cycle of your hair, which is two to five years long. However, split ends *will* slow down the rate at which hair grows, so cutting them is important in maintaining normal growth.

Myth:
Many mothers think that a child's hair will grow in thicker if it is cut often.

Fact:
Hair texture has nothing to do with frequency of cutting—it's what nature has given you. However, a child's hair, which often has a very fine and silky texture, will give the illusion of being thicker when the fine ends are cut.

Myth:
If you shampoo too often, you will weaken the hair.

Fact:
Wet hair is more vulnerable to breakage because of improper detangling, but that is not the point about shampooing: You shampoo your hair to keep it clean and healthy looking, not to weaken it.

Myth:
If you shampoo too often or even every day, your hair will become oily.

Fact:
It is just the reverse. Oily hair *should* be shampooed every day.

Myth:
When hair is split at the ends, the splits will travel all the way down to the roots.

Fact:
Split ends don't travel. Regular cutting and shaping of the hair will end split ends by getting rid of them. The use of a conditioner after each shampoo and a deep treatment once in a while will keep them from getting worse.

Myth:
Pregnant women's hair will not take any chemical processes well (permanent waving, coloring, or streaking, for instance).

Fact:
Chemical processes done to the hair are not affected by the hormonal balance of an expectant mother. In fact, hair reacts very well when a woman is pregnant. And what better time is there for her to try to look and feel even more beautiful?

23

Myth:	Fact:
Conditioners will make curly hair curlier.	Conditioners can only add shine, fluff, and softness to already existing curls. Curly hair is something you are born with. It is a structural condition and not at all affected by applied conditioners (which don't penetrate the hair anyway).
If you pull out one gray hair, five more will grow in its place.	Only one hair at a time grows from a single hair follicle.
Permanent waving will cause dandruff.	Dandruff is an oily scalp condition and has nothing to do with the chemical process of permanent waving.
If you wash your hair every day, you will take all the natural oils out.	Shampoos today are pH-balanced, which means they are specially formulated not to strip the hair of its natural oils.
If you keep having your hair chemically straightened, it will eventually become straight by itself.	Straightening affects only the hair already on your head—not any new hair that will grow in.
If you have your hair permed consistently, it will become naturally curly.	Permanent waving will curl only the hair to which the chemical is applied—not hair that has yet to emerge.
If you blow-dry your hair a great deal, it will get naturally straighter.	The more you blow-dry, the more damage you might do to your hair. Nature, not drying technique, determines straight hair.
When hair reaches a certain length, it will stop growing.	Hair growth is ongoing. There is a stage, however, when hair reaches maturity, after which the growth rate is minimal. This may lead you to believe it has stopped growing. But it hasn't. Also, the growth of long hair is not as perceptible as the growth of short hair.

Myth:	Fact:
Hair grows from the ends.	Just the reverse is true. Growth starts from the root, which is several layers under the scalp.
Coloring the hair will eventually alter the natural pigmentation.	Chemical processes alter only the hair that's on the head. The new growth will come back with your natural pigmentation. If the opposite were true, you would never need retouching!
My mother had gray hair early, so I guess I will too.	Early graying seems to be hereditary. However, this is not a proven scientific fact.
Gray hair comes from tension.	Gray hair comes from a loss of natural pigmentations. There have been some cases of people turning "white from fright," but there is no scientific explanation for this phenomenon.
You should not shampoo your hair until two weeks after having had a permanent wave or a straightening.	Shampoo will not interfere with the effects of a chemical processing. Nor will it damage the hair. You can shampoo within 24 hours after having had these treatments.
Permanent waving will remove all the oil on my scalp and hair.	Perms will curl the hair, not remove scalp oil. Oil on the scalp is a question of hormones and diet. However, excessive use of chemicals can dry out and damage hair and scalp.
Hair grows in better if cut when the moon is full.	Hair grows by its own timetable. A full moon won't affect hair growth!
Don't have your hair cut when you're sick, because it won't look or hang as well as when you are well.	Illness can dull the hair, but a good haircut looks good no matter what.

History and myth, fact and fiction. Where does one stop and the other start? I hope I've armed you with enough information to help you sort it all out—because knowing the facts about your hair, understanding its real nature, is the first step on the way to beautiful, healthy, easy-to-care-for hair.

nutrition

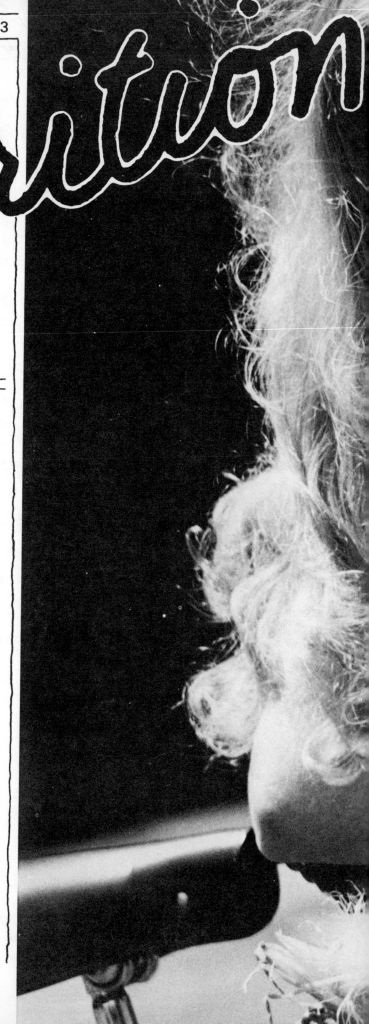

We carry around about 100,000 hairs on our head at any one time, and though that may sound like a mind-boggling quantity, we never seem to be bothered by this weightless burden except when it doesn't look good or starts to fall out. But we are always losing some hair and growing new hair. It is a normal process. In some sense it is an extraordinary process, since each hair is an individual and has nothing to do with its neighbor.

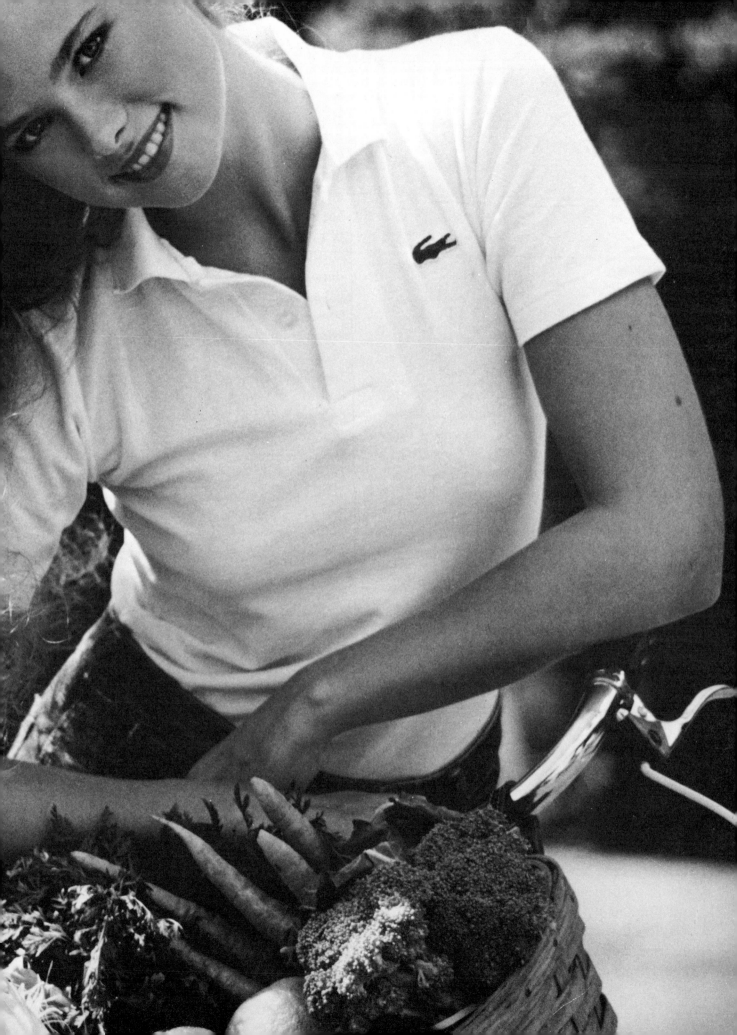

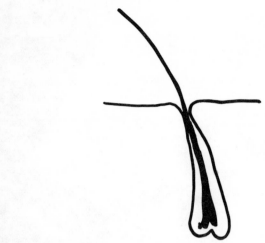

WHAT IS HAIR?

Located in the dermis, that layer of skin lower than the outer epidermis on your head, is the papilla—a very small bud at the base of the hair follicle. The hair bulb, or root, is formed in the papilla, or base, and becomes firmly attached over it. Small blood vessels carry the ingredients needed to form hair to the papilla, where they are changed into keratin. Keratin, in turn, forms hair. A type of protein, keratin is made up of a complex combination of amino acids. There are twenty-one known amino acids which are responsible for the structure of protein. Ten of these cannot be manufactured by the body, and must be had from outside sources. So the formation of keratin is dependent on specific ingredients being carried by the bloodstream to the papilla, and many of these are supplied by the food we eat. This is why diet and nutrition are so important for the growth and health of hair. Keratin is a tough, elastic material: When it forms continuous sheets, fingernails are created; when it forms long fibers, the result is hair.

The long keratin fibers that make up a hair's structure are actually long molecular chains wound around each other in a ropelike manner and bonded by various elements including hydrogen, cystine, and sulfur. These not only stabilize a hair's structure, but lend it physical properties such as body, strength, and elasticity.

Hair Growth. Waiting for hair and nails to grow sometimes feels as agonizing as watching water come to a boil. It's endless. But believe it or not, there's a lot of activity and growing going on on our heads all the time. Hair usually grows approximately .3 to .4 millimeters a day. The entire growth cycle lasts somewhere between two and five years, during which time the hair produces tremendous amounts of protein. This is called the "anagen" stage. After the fifth year, something shuts down the growth. The hair goes into a brief "catagen" stage, which lasts a week or two. Then it slides into a resting phase—the "telogen" stage. This period lasts only a few months, at which point the old hair is pushed out by new hair and the cycle starts again.

Hair Structure. If you were to examine a cross section of a single hair under a microscope, you would see that it has three distinct layers:

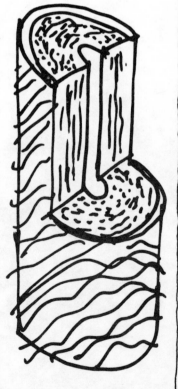

The cuticle is the outermost layer, which consists of hard, flat scales that overlap one another like roof shingles. This overlapping arrangement provides protection for the cortex and at the same time gives strength and flexibility to the hair. It is the cuticle's flexibility that lets our hair be waved, curled, twisted, or braided without breaking. When hair is in good condition, the cuticle scales will lie flat, creating a smooth, reflective surface against which light can bounce. This is what shiny hair is all about. When hair is damaged and unhealthy, the cuticle scales break off and their edges become ragged. This uneven surface no longer mirrors light and causes hair to look dull, drab, and lifeless.

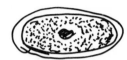 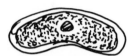

The cortex is the layer immediately below the outer cuticle, and it makes up about 75 to 90 percent of the hair's bulk. Many of the physical properties attributed to keratin in general are characteristics of the cortex. In the cortex the fibrous, ropelike structure of hair (keratin) is most evident. It is this fibrous inner core that gives hair its strength, elasticity, and pliability. Pigment (hair color) is also produced within the cortex, and this important layer governs other hair properties such as direction of growth, size and diameter of hair strands, and texture and quality. Many experts feel that the natural wave in the hair is determined by the shape the cortex takes while the hair is being formed in the follicle. In the cross sections of hair showing the shape of the cortex, look at the difference between straight, wavy, and curly hair. Straight hair has a circular cortex, while that of wavy and curly hair is more oval and elongated. When you want to change the hair's natural form with either perms or relaxers, the chemicals must penetrate and change the structure of the cortex.

The medulla is the innermost layer of hair and its function is really unknown. The medulla may even be completely absent—although its absence doesn't seem to affect the individual hair shaft in any way.

Hair Type. Once you know what hair *is,* you can start trying to understand the kind you've got. The first step toward great-looking hair is to categorize your own hair's individual texture, curl factor, oil level, and condition.

Texture. The diameter of the hair determines its texture—and this varies greatly even among the hairs on a single head.

Fine hair usually has a very small and narrow diameter. The hair strands tend to look limp and lack body.

Medium hair is just what the name implies—somewhere between the narrow, fine hair strand and the fatter, coarse strand.

Coarse hair is characterized by strong, almost wiry fibers. Its diameter is much larger than that of fine hair.

Curl Factor. Know your curl factor or wave pattern. Whether hair is straight, wavy, curly, or frizzy is determined by the way the keratin forms within the cortex. Wave patterns can vary not only from strand to strand, but within the same strand: A single hair can have a combination of patterns.

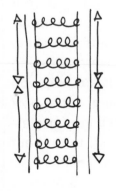 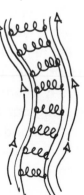 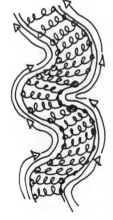

Oil Level. Your hair is lubricated and nourished by oil secreted from sebaceous glands next to your hair follicles, and the amount of oil the scalp produces very often is related to the body's hormonal condition. At certain stages during your life when hormones are extremely active, you will tend to produce more oil. The oil production will taper off as you get older.

Oily hair is actually an oily scalp condition usually caused by overactive sebaceous glands. It is the scalp that secretes the oil, not the hair. The oil travels down the hair shaft to create oily hair.

Dry hair is usually hair that has been stripped of its natural oils through excessive use of chemicals, processing, sun and weather extremes, or underactive sebaceous glands. It can also "look" dry if the cuticle has been damaged by chemicals, teasing, improper brushing, and so on. Because of this damage light cannot be reflected, and so the hair will seem dry and dull.

Combination oily/dry hair most often manifests itself in an oily scalp with bone-dry hair ends. While the sebaceous glands continue to produce oil through the scalp, the hair shaft can lose its moisture from any number of causes, such as excessive blow-drying and chemical processing.

Condition. Evaluate your hair condition and damage and learn its cause (mechanical, chemical, weather, etc.). Only you can analyze your beauty regimen to see if you are, for example, blow-drying with a very high heat setting, baking in the sun for hours on end, or overprocessing your hair with too many chemicals. To help you spot trouble, try plucking out a single strand of hair. Pull it firmly on both ends, testing for elasticity and stretch. Almost everything else about your hair is related to this: Strong, healthy hair has resilience and will stretch up to 25 percent without breaking. Dry, brittle, lifeless hair will break and snap immediately.

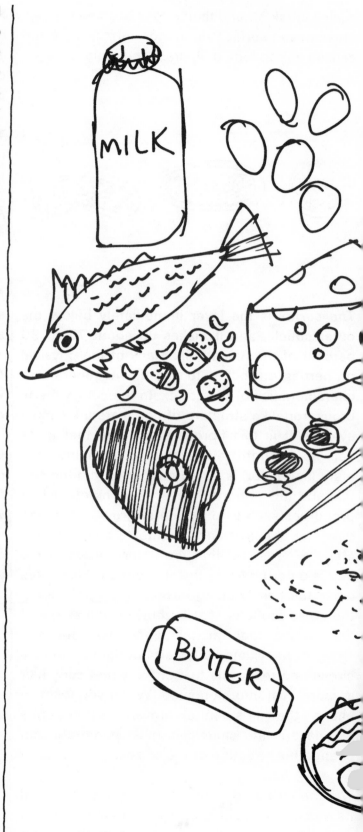

HAIR AND NUTRITION

Since what we eat affects the growth, quality, and health of our hair, it is important to understand how the vitamin and mineral content of certain foods works. But a little knowledge can be dangerous in this area, because all too often food facts turn into food fads with the result that scores of people storm the vitamin counters to pop improper dosages of both vitamins and minerals. It is a proven fact that the whole nutritional network is like a giant spiderweb. If one thread is pulled, the whole web becomes distorted. So it is extremely important to understand the balance and interrelationship between vitamins and minerals and our bodies—including our hair. Since there are many excellent books on the subject (one of the most popular being *Let's Eat Right to Keep Fit* by nutrition expert Adelle Davis), I want only to highlight a few of the most vital nutritional aids to healthy hair here.

Protein. The production of hair requires that the diet include a constant supply of high-grade protein. Lean meat, fish, eggs, cheese, and milk are good sources. Adelle Davis said, "Since hair and nails are made of protein, this nutrient must be adequate to maintain their health."

The American diet is rich in protein, sometimes too rich. For example, a woman needs 46 grams of protein a day on the average, and that amounts to less than 2 ounces. A man needs about 56 grams, or just 2 ounces. In fact, however, the average American diet provides about 100 grams a day. What happens when you take in extra protein? You either use it up as energy or store it as fat. So extra protein doesn't mean extra protein for your hair. It could mean simply extra fat around your tummy!

Vitamin A. Again, most Americans get ample vitamin A in fish, liver, butter, whole milk, eggs, and cheese. In addition, adequate supplies of it are stored in the liver. When we get enough vitamin A, it helps give us healthy skin and hair. When it is undersupplied, the hair becomes dry and lacks luster. But too much vitamin A can be toxic and actually causes hair loss. So maintaining a proper nutritional balance is important.

Copper. A deficiency of this mineral can cause depigmentation of hair (graying). Foods rich in copper are raisins, nuts, and liver. Also, copper is easily obtained, in part, from foods cooked in copper utensils.

Zinc. There is a high concentration of zinc in hair. A deficiency of this mineral can cause roughening of the skin and even hair loss. Grain and wheat products are good sources of zinc. And if you feel extravagant, oysters are tremendously rich in zinc. Processed and refined foods, however, are very poor sources. By the way, if you are taking birth control pills or if you are pregnant, your body may require additional zinc.

Crash Diets. Any food regimen that severely alters the nutritional balance and deprives the body of protein will affect hair. In some cases the growth rate will slow down significantly and can even result in hair loss. Other hair problems can occur during dieting, ranging from dull and scruffy-looking hair to severe hair fall-out.

In addition to vitamins and diet, other internal functions and external factors play a major role in the health and growth of hair.

HAIR AND HORMONES

Hormonal imbalances or disorders can create hair loss. An overproduction of androgen, a male hormone, will cause loss of hair *or* hair growth, and testosterone can lead to temporary balding. A deficiency of adrenal hormones can also cause some loss of hair.

And thyroid hormones affect hair. A deficiency will result in hair loss and an excess will result in the hair becoming extremely fine and silky.

HAIR AND DRUGS

Hair growth depends on an actively dividing cell structure. Whenever a drug interferes with cell division, it will affect hair. For example, in chemotherapy, the anticancer drugs interfere with cell proliferation and cell division, causing severe hair loss. Birth control pills and other drugs that affect hormonal balance will also affect hair, since hair growth is very much dependent on the body's hormonal structure.

HAIR AND STRESS

There is as yet no conclusive scientific documentation for connecting hair loss and stress. But there are proposed theories that say an increase in the flow of adrenaline can cause the small blood vessels to constrict, which in turn might constrict the hair follicle enough to cause it to atrophy and die.

But even without scientific proof, we do know that stress and trauma have an effect on our bodies, especially with respect to color change. Don't we "turn white with fright" or "red with rage"? The interrelationships that exist within the body are intricate, and perhaps one day we'll have all the answers to the questions. In the meantime, we know that stress takes its toll on lots of things, including our hair.

HAIR CARE RECIPES

Now that you've read all about your body's nutritional needs and how they affect hair, you're probably ready to learn some "external" ways by which you can give your hair a boost. I have been creating—or should I say "concocting"—recipes for the hair for many years. They're for fighting dullness, controlling oiliness, adding highlights, for conditioning all kinds of textures, and on and on, and they're all fully described later on, in the appropriate chapters. Most of the ingredients can be purchased at your local vegetable market, health food shop, or drugstore. They're fun and easy to whip up. But even though many of them look delicious enough to eat or drink, *don't!* They are to be applied to the hair externally and not ingested.

Hair Loss. As I said earlier, we are always losing hair as part of the natural growth cycle. Hair loss from pathological causes is a broad field of study with many answers still to be found. For example, certain diseases cause hair loss because they are said to speed up the hair's growth cycle. Instead of a hair taking the normal two to five years to mature in the anagen stage, this time span can be speeded up to just a few months so that the hair enters "old age" in a relatively short time.

Clinical studies have shown that excessive loss of hair during the anagen, or growing, stage can be caused by X-ray treatment, overprocessing in styling, trauma, infectious disease, metabolic and endocrine disorders, or prolonged pressure on the scalp, to mention a few.

In the same studies hair loss during the telogen (resting) stage was attributed to stress, crash diets, surgery, anesthesia, and other causes.

RINSE RECIPES (See Chapter 9, **Conditioners**)

- *SPEARMINT RINSE for shine and controlling oiliness*
- *EUCALPYTUS RINSE for shine and controlling oiliness*
- *CUCUMBER RINSE for oily hair*
- *LEMON JUICE RINSE for shine*
- *CAMOMILE RINSE for blonde hair*
- *THYME RINSE for dandruff*
- *ROSEMARY RINSE for dull hair*
- *SAGE RINSE for oily hair*

CONDITIONER AND TREATMENT RECIPES (See Chapter 9, **Conditioners**)

- *MAYONNAISE CONDITIONER for dry hair*
- *MAYONNAISE AND EGG CONDITIONER for dry and coarse hair*
- *WATERCRESS TREATMENT for oily hair*
- *YEAST CURE for problem hair*
- *FLOUR PASTE for frizzy hair*
- *POMADE for frizzy hair*
- *INSTANT EGG CONDITIONER for dry, tired hair*
- *BEEF MARROW TREATMENT for dry, damaged hair*
- *VITAMIN E TREATMENT for damaged hair*

SETTING LOTION RECIPES (See Chapter 11, **Setting**)

- *SUGAR WATER*
- *RICE WATER*

COLOR RECIPES (See Chapter 12, **Coloring**)

FOR LIGHT HAIR
- *Beach Boy Color*
- *Henna Flash*
- *Color Whip*
- *Lemon and Lime Swizzle*
- *Lemon Squeeze*

FOR LIGHT TO MEDIUM-BROWN HAIR
- *Avocado Lightener*
- *Herbal Pack*
- *Henna Streak*

FOR LIGHT OR RED HAIR
- *Sun Glow*

FOR DARK AND AUBURN HAIR
- *Blackberry Cocktail*
- *Henna Espresso*

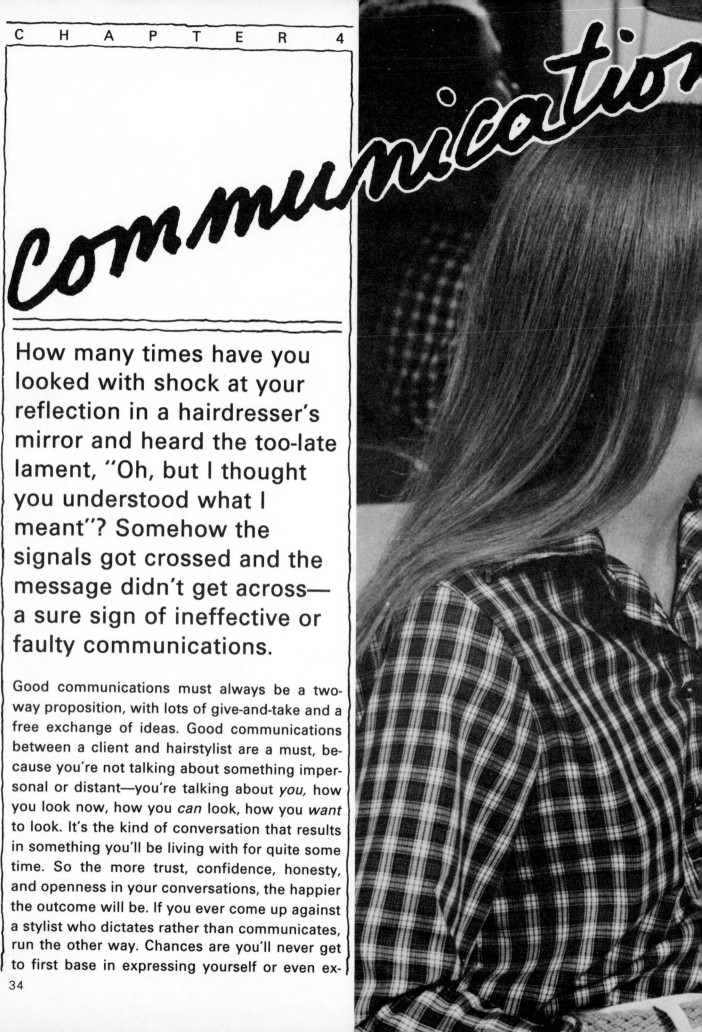

CHAPTER 4

Communication

How many times have you looked with shock at your reflection in a hairdresser's mirror and heard the too-late lament, "Oh, but I thought you understood what I meant"? Somehow the signals got crossed and the message didn't get across— a sure sign of ineffective or faulty communications.

Good communications must always be a two-way proposition, with lots of give-and-take and a free exchange of ideas. Good communications between a client and hairstylist are a must, because you're not talking about something impersonal or distant—you're talking about *you*, how you look now, how you *can* look, how you *want* to look. It's the kind of conversation that results in something you'll be living with for quite some time. So the more trust, confidence, honesty, and openness in your conversations, the happier the outcome will be. If you ever come up against a stylist who dictates rather than communicates, run the other way. Chances are you'll never get to first base in expressing yourself or even ex-

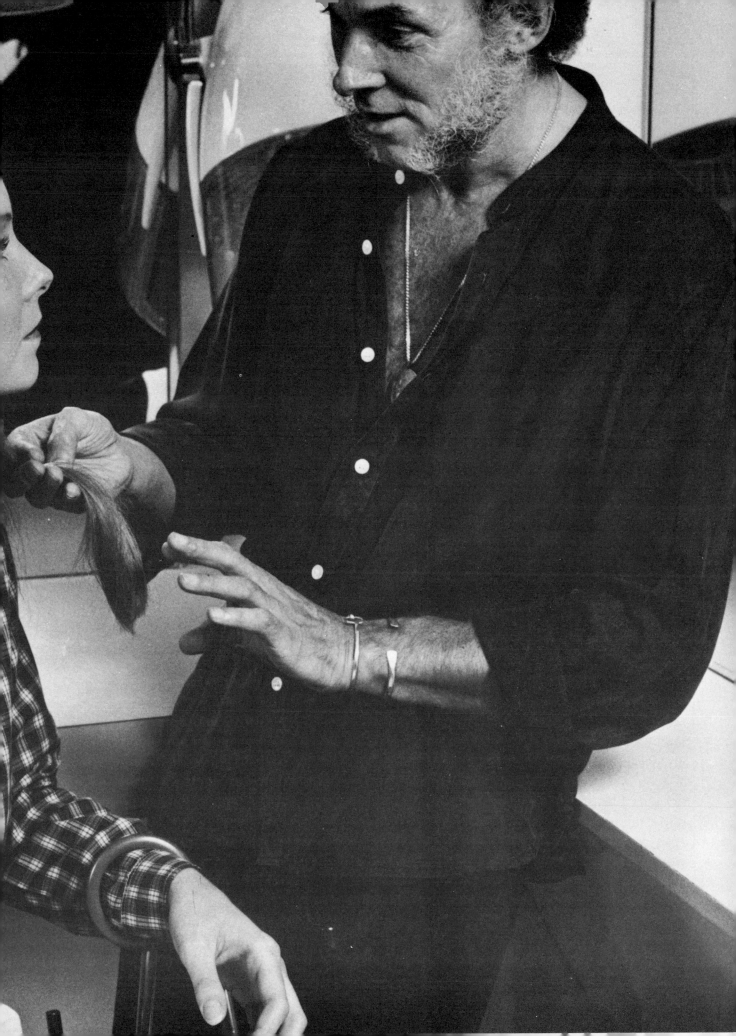

ploring what you want, because that kind of closed-minded stylist will never be interested in what *you* have to say.

Why Communicate? Any change in your appearance—especially one you can't control—is unsettling. Having long hair shortened, dark hair lightened, or straight hair curled can be a frightening and overwhelming experience for many women, because there is always the possibility that the change will be disastrous. Talking about it beforehand with a stylist or colorist can do wonders in minimizing those fears, and in reassuring that you will get the look you want.

Good communications can also help you evaluate what kinds of changes, if any, you really do want to make. Every good stylist or colorist must play the role of psychiatrist from time to time. For instance, a client walks in depressed and frustrated and wants a drastic change, thinking "another image" might make the difference between feeling blue and feeling better. The stylist, who has seen this behavior pattern before, knows that in a day or two she'll feel different and hate the change (and probably the stylist, too, who "let" her make the switch). My approach to the problem would be to stop it before it becomes one. I would try to discourage or explore the client's radical ideas and suggest that if she's determined to make a major change she must ask herself these questions: Why do I want the change? Is it someone else's idea or my own? Have I given it enough thought or is it a spur-of-the-moment decision? Interestingly enough, flash changes tend to happen most often after the Christmas holidays when the tinsel's packed away, the festivities are over, the weather is getting colder, and excitement seems increasingly difficult to find. Underneath the mountain of hats, gloves, and sweaters, there is usually a woman yearning to escape the boredom of the long winter months ahead. She thinks a new hair color or cut or style will do the

trick. My advice: Please proceed with caution. These are the *worst* times to contemplate a major change in your appearance. Don't make a hasty decision that you'll regret later! Acknowledge those restless feelings, and then sit down and talk openly with your stylist or colorist about what you'd like to change. If you've been able to establish good communications, he or she can guide you in the right direction. During this period, don't expect your hairdresser to change your life-style along with your hairstyle. A new, flattering look is never a cure for loneliness, boredom, or a cold winter, even though it can give your ego a substantial boost.

SELECTING THE RIGHT SALON AND STYLIST

Selecting the appropriate salon and finding the right stylist are, of course, the first steps in the communication process. A lot of women don't even know how to start. One of the easiest and most direct ways of finding a good salon and stylist is by *asking*. If you see someone with a terrific haircut or color, don't hesitate to inquire where it was done, who did it, and how much it cost. Or you can start your search by reading the beauty and fashion magazines. Often finding the salon for you is a simple matter of reading the photo credits or calling the beauty editor of a magazine. But remember that hair fashions come and go, and publications covering them will show what's new on the market—not necessarily what's right for *you*. Choosing the look that fits you and your life is up to you. So investigate. Gather inspiration wherever you can. But make the final decision yourself.

Once you have selected a few salons to test, make an appointment for a consultation. This service is often free. Try to see the salon owner, who is usually the most experienced staff member and knows the precise talents of each of his operators. Every new client represents a new challenge, and if the salon owner is really good he'll be excited about talking with you and helping. So don't be afraid to go for a consultation and ask as many questions as you like. If you feel you're getting a brush-off instead of a consultation, that's a hint that this is not the salon for you. While you're at the shop, look around. Do you like the work that's being done? Does the atmosphere of the shop blend with your personality? Is the clientele within your age group? All these checkpoints add up to a total picture of the right salon for you.

The Mother-Daughter Mistake. One mistake to avoid if you're the daughter of a mother with a favorite beauty salon is being influenced by what "Mother thinks best." I have seen over and over a mother's image of herself pushed onto her daughter. Too many times mothers like to see their offspring look like them without ever considering the age difference. Even more disastrous are those mothers who try to influence the hairdresser into cutting the daughter's hair a certain length or style—a look that doesn't suit daughter at all, but rather suits mother because she has hers done that way. Too many times, I hate to admit, hairdressers listen to Mom, never

taking into consideration the younger woman's age, features, hair texture, life-style, and the more important fact that most daughters really don't *want* to be carbon copies of their mothers. My suggestion to all daughters: Don't be swayed by your mother's advice. Try turning the tables instead, and get her to use *your* hairstylist!

Ask Questions. At your consultation, ask as many questions as necessary to make you feel at ease. If you lack confidence in your stylist or colorist, chances are you'll never be happy or comfortable with the results. Tell him or her exactly what you want so you can avoid the sad tales of mistakes later on. There is nothing wrong with showing your hair to your stylist before you have anything done to it, if you think that is the only way to communicate. Show it while it's dry to make sure the stylist sees, firsthand, your degree of curl, frizz, straightness, etc. Tell the stylist whether you've washed it recently, how you dried it, and how you set it or styled it. After the first visit, he or she should know your hair and understand how it reacts. If you continue showing the stylist your hair at every visit, it indicates a lack of confidence on your part in the

---

Checklist for Selecting a Salon

☐ Receptionist's attitude (Is she or he snobby, friendly, attentive, distracted?)

☐ Comfort of waiting area (Enough seating, magazines?)

☐ Kind of music being played (Is it rock or classical, or is it the news? Is it loud, blaring, or soft?)

☐ Decor (Is it formal or casual? Does it make you feel out of place?)

☐ Staff interaction (Are they cooperative, argumentative, too self-involved?)

☐ Age of clientele (Do you feel they're all old enough to be your mother, or do they make *you* feel like a grandmother?)

☐ Type of products for sale (Does the shop look more like a department store than a hair salon? Are non-hair-related items being sold, and if so, at what price?)

☐ Degree of pressure to buy goods or services

☐ Type of work being done (Watch for a prevalence of old-fashioned styles, use of hair spray, teasing, extensive use of rollers.)

☐ Type of equipment used (Is it primarily old-fashioned, up-to-date?)

☐ Ease with which you get a consultation

☐ Quality of consultant (How would you rate his or her patience, interest, understanding?)

☐ Prices

stylist. And that's not fair to either of you. If you're not sure what you want, bring a picture of a look you like and this will help the stylist to understand what you have in mind. If you can't find a photo of something you like and haven't a clue as to what look you feel you should have, you'll have to trust the stylist with the decision. If you still have doubts, say so. It's your hair, and you must live with it—not the stylist. If the stylist or colorist acts impatient when you ask questions or doesn't explain a decision or your personalities clash, make the change to another person pronto and avoid future trouble.

COMMUNICATIONS AND COLOR

If you are considering a color change, there are a few special points you should discuss with your colorist. First, what will the final look be? If the change is drastic, brunette to blonde, for instance, are you ready for it emotionally? If you really believe you are and that the change will give you a psychological lift, proceed full steam ahead! Also think about the retouching necessary for color upkeep. How often will you need to return for touch-ups? Can you afford them? And

what about the effect of chemicals on your hair? Can the quality and texture of your hair take such potential abuse? And what about the treatments or conditioners necessary to compensate for chemical damage? Are you willing to spend the time, effort, and money to keep your hair healthy? There are always pros and cons to using chemicals, so weigh them carefully before trying them—not after it's too late.

It's also very important to tell your colorist before the coloring process starts (no matter whether it's full color or highlighting) if you have already had any other chemical treatments done to your hair, such as permanent waving, straightening, etc. These can affect the success of the color application, and so the operator should be fully aware of what he or she is dealing with. In the end, this will prevent complications, and the results will be that much better.

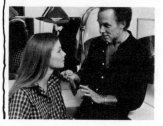

Checklist for Communicating with the Colorist

- ☐ Bring a swatch or picture of the color you like to help the colorist understand your preferences.
- ☐ Discuss eye and skin tone. These are the basis for the perfect choice of hair color.
- ☐ Discuss the original color of your hair, especially if it's processed.
- ☐ Tell the colorist what you have used on your hair (henna, relaxers, perms, etc.).
- ☐ Go to the same shop for coloring and styling because color-processed hair requires special handling and understanding.

- ☐ Discuss the use of special hair care products and treatments with the colorist (shampoos, conditioners, blow-drying, rollers, etc.).
- ☐ Be sure the colorist understands your life-style and time availability. This affects return visits for touch-ups, etc.
- ☐ Discuss prices and the cost of monthly upkeep before any coloring is done.
- ☐ Be sure the colorist's personality suits you.
- ☐ Don't be afraid to switch to someone better.

COMMUNICATIONS AND HAIR CARE

A good stylist should always discuss what cut will enhance your face shape and how much time you normally spend on hair care. If you're the wash-and-wear type (a person who wants to spend the least amount of time and effort on her hair), you won't be happy crowned with rollers. Your hairstyle should reflect your personality. But please understand that sometimes what you prefer or project is virtually impossible because of your hair's texture and quality. There's no point, for instance, in dreaming about fabulously curly locks when yours are arrow-straight and baby-fine. Remember, try doing what's best for you with what you've already got. Pushing your hair into a look that won't work will only cause unnecessary frustration.

One important question you must ask yourself—and discuss with your stylist—is how handy you are with hair tools. You might look fantastic as you step outside the beauty salon, but that image isn't worth much unless you're capable of achieving the same look by yourself. So ask for some tips on styling at home between shampoos. I am a firm believer in helping the client learn how to handle her own hair more effectively. For example, if you just can't get the hang of handling a blow-dryer, switch to one of my natural setting methods (see Chapter 11). A good stylist should make suggestions about what brush to use, how to brush the hair, how to use accessories such as combs, barrettes, etc. Anything that can add to a woman's look and make her life easier should come in the form of "free advice" from a stylist.

Once good communications have been established, you'll be amazed at how much freer, easier, and more relaxed you'll be in that salon chair. Remember, your confidence triggers the hairdresser's creativity. Your belief in his or her talent sparks their potential—and yours.

Tipping. How much and who to tip can cause embarrassing moments for some clients. My rule of thumb is to tip those people who work on your hair the same percentage you would use for a good waiter or waitress—15 to 20 percent of the charge for that particular service—but if a salon *owner* does your hair, no tipping is necessary.

Checklist for Communicating with the Stylist

☐ Take pictures of a look you like—especially if you're not sure what you want.

☐ Learn the buzzwords in haircutting. A "health cut" takes a ¼" off all around to get rid of split ends. A "shaping" is the same as a "trim"—an average 1" cut all around, not more.

☐ Expect your stylist to listen as well as talk.

☐ Expect your stylist to discuss your face shape, hair texture, and hair type with you before ever picking up the scissors, helping you understand the potential of your hair—what you can expect or not expect it to do.

☐ Tell the stylist about any previous treatments, especially any chemical processing.

☐ Expect your stylist to explain clearly when you should come back for a shaping or restyling.

☐ Make sure you're told how to take care of your hair by yourself at home.

☐ Expect your stylist to tell you what products you should be using and what you should avoid.

☐ Feel free to ask *any* question that occurs to you, no matter how silly or ignorant you think it sounds.

☐ Don't be afraid to switch stylists within the same shop.

☐ Both parties should understand each other completely before any work is done.

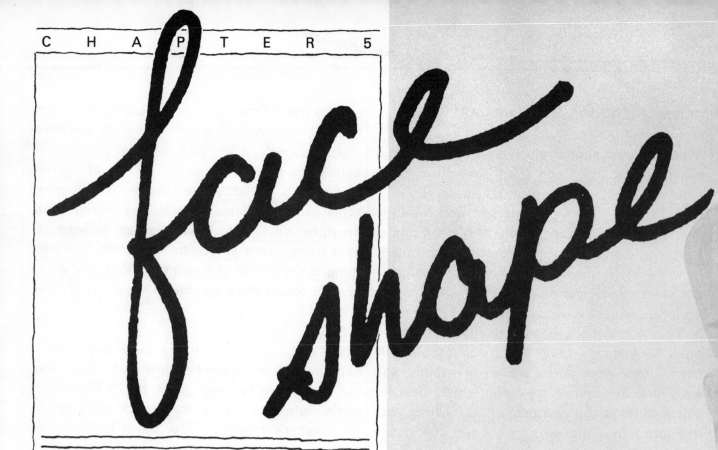

face shape

Faces are personalities. Not cookie-cutter components. Or mirror images of geometric shapes (squares, triangles, circles, etc.). If that's all they were, we'd find ourselves at the architect's office each week instead of the beauty salon. I know that there are experts in my business who constantly try to package looks into tidy little bundles so they'll fit a mold. But I refuse to believe we're assembly-line products. We are people. Full of style, character, and differences. And fortunately, our faces

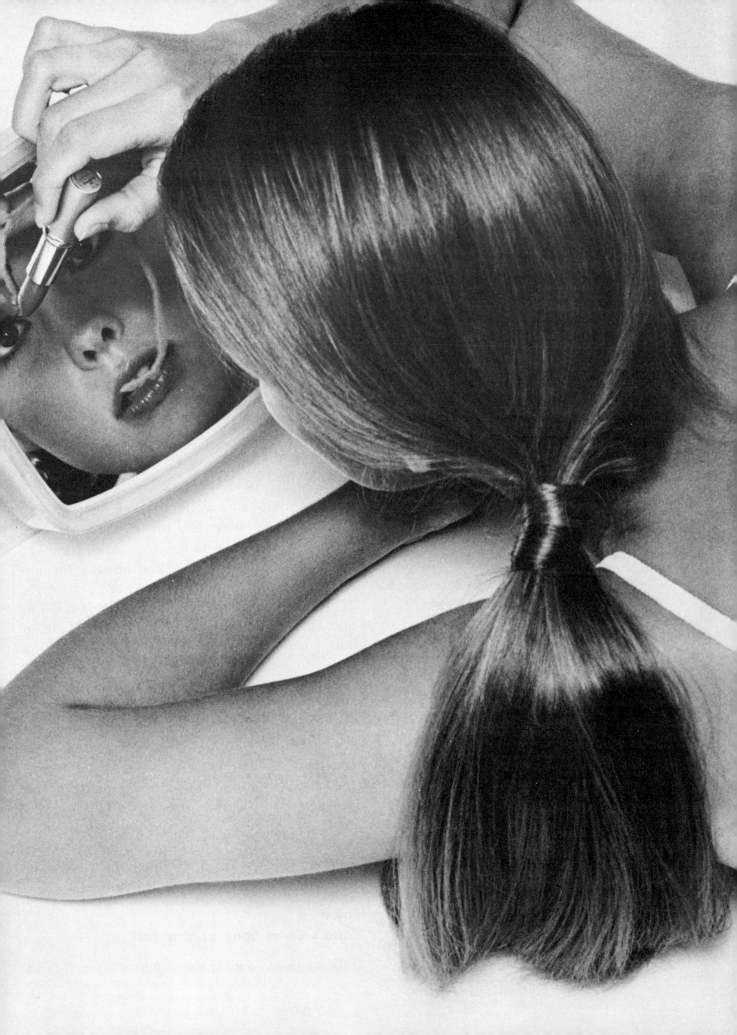

have millions of wonderful variations. That's what makes them interesting to look at, to explore, to change, to capture in photography, to keep in lockets, to fall in love with.

That faces *can* be classified by their basic shapes is true, but this is only so we can have easy reference points and guidelines to work with. Faces can never be considered absolutely oval, or square, or triangular, or round. That's why the tips I'm going to give you now are not meant to be hard-and-fast rules and can be broken successfully. They are not gospel. What's even more important is that if you are comfortable with your features as they are, keep on doing whatever you're doing—whether or not the way you wear your hair is "right" for your shape face. On the other hand, if you want to de-emphasize, play up, or get around some special problem, you'll find some fresh ideas about how to make an easy change for the better.

Here are a few points I would like to underscore.

The first point:
Your Face Is Not an Island.

Rather, it is part of your overall proportions, and must be considered that way. The same is true of your hair. It is an integral part of your face, yet more than face shape is involved when cutting and shaping it. For example, when I look at a client I don't put her in a precise "face-shape box" and leave her there. Her features may be large or small, even or uneven. Her neck may be short or long (and length of neck is very important, since it's the pedestal for the head). Her shoulders may be wide or narrow. She may be tall, thin, heavy, or short. In other words, her face does not exist

by itself and shouldn't be isolated from the rest of her body. It's part of a bigger picture. If it is treated as a separate entity, she could easily wind up like many other very tall, large-featured, big-boned women with hair too short. It isn't until you see her standing that you realize the lack of balance between her hair and the rest of her body. In this case, the result would be a very unattractive "pinhead look."

I have seen lots of other disasters that even an Army "lawn-mower cut" couldn't match. This is why I will *never* cut a client's hair without having her first stand up in front of a full-length mirror. I want to see her proportions in perspective so that everything will work together. And so that the cut will be *her* cut and not a textbook shape (see Chapter 6).

The second point:
Break the Rules.

Rules in the beauty world are meant to be bent, if not broken. After all, the hemline dictums seem to have gone out the window. Now we wear what pleases us ... and not the fashion world. There are already so many dos and don'ts in life and love that I certainly wouldn't want to add any when it comes to having great-looking hair. I can't stress that enough. If you like the way you look, if you've invested in creating a style you are happy with and identify with, forget about the "better" way! For example, not every woman with a high forehead wants to minimize it with bangs. She may like her high forehead and think it signifies intelligence, insight, and special character. So bangs for her are out of the question, and I would never try to talk her into them, any more than I would advise Katharine Hepburn to cut her hair to soften her strikingly square jawline. That's her signature. That's the way she wants to look. That's her self-image.

The third point:
Take a Good Look at Yourself.

Self-image has a lot to do with how honestly and

openly you see yourself. Part of developing self-image is knowing all about the basic guidelines and how to apply them. That's precisely what gives you the ammunition to ignore the rules successfully, *if* you want to. A good starting point is being able to look in the mirror and see yourself objectively. Know your pluses and minuses. Evaluate your good points. Experiment with ways to play them up. Find your weak spots and learn the ways to minimize them (or accentuate them if that's what you prefer). One other important tip to remember is that camouflage doesn't always solve a problem. Sometimes it puts it in the spotlight.

Now let's begin with the first step:

HOW TO FIND YOUR OWN FACE SHAPE

You'd be amazed at how few women know what category their face shape fits, especially when they usually know their exact dress size or their exact shade of lipstick or rouge. So here's a quick and easy way to find out what shape your face really is . . . or isn't. You need only three props: a scarf, a mirror, a lipstick or felt-tip marker. Here's what you do.

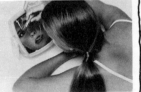

1. Wrap the scarf around your head and tie it so it pulls the hair back off your face. 2. Stand 12" from the mirror. 3. With one eye closed, use the lipstick to draw the outline of your face as you see it, on the mirror. You don't have to be the least bit artistic to do this. And don't worry—the lipstick or marker comes off with a little window cleaner. 4. Look at the shape you've drawn and compare it to one of the six basic shapes shown in this chapter.

Remember, your face won't be an exact duplicate of any single shape because no face ever is. But it will probably come closer to one shape than any other.

Once you've determined what shape face you've got, you can then experiment with some of the hair tricks I have devised over the years. Also, you'll learn some pointers about my basic cut, because with variations—differences in length or the same length all around, changes in the part, bangs or no bangs, ends turned up or under, angled higher or lower in back—this is the cut that will work for every shape of face.

These face-shape guidelines apply whether your hair is straight or curly, just as long as you understand the direction of its movement. If your hair is curly, remember that curls give more volume—be careful to use your curls for softness and fullness or they might come out looking too wild. My feature-balancing tips will also work whether your hair is layered or blunt-cut. But don't make the common mistake of believing that by layering your hair you are adding fullness and bounce. You are not. In fact, cutting hair in layers takes away volume and can often leave your head looking flat. Layered hair needs body for height or fullness. A permanent wave means you won't have to fuss as much. If you're looking for fullness, you're better off with a blunt cut and it's easier to handle than a layered cut when you are trying to balance features.

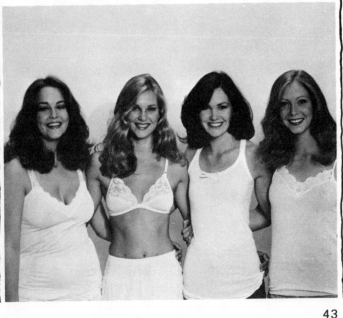

1 The Square Face.

The Square Face. This face shape is usually characterized by an angular jaw and a square brow. Most of the tips that follow will help soften the sharp angle of the jawline and minimize the squared-off brow. (However, if you want to maximize the square look, play it to the hilt . . . do just the opposite.)

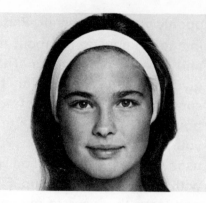

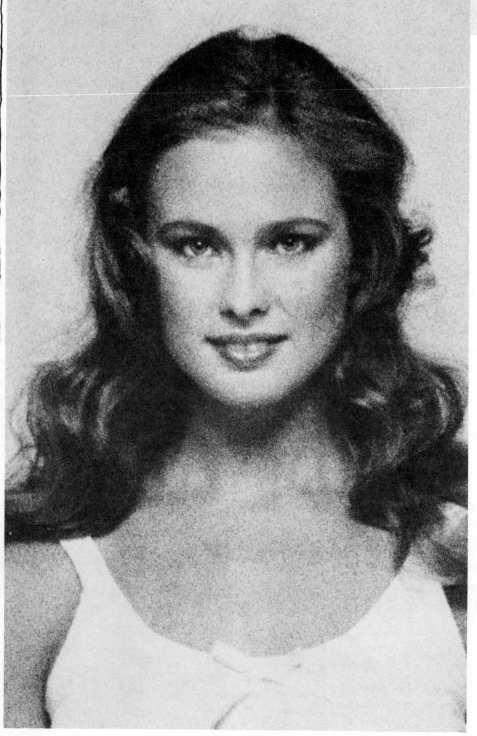

1. Wear hair swinging forward on the face. This cuts the angle of the jaw. If the hair is cut slightly shorter in back, the forward swing will happen naturally.

2. Try an off-center part. It will soften the square angle of the brow.

3. Wear hair on the forehead. It's the perfect softener. It can be a "curtain" of hair cut wispy in the middle so that it falls naturally and gradually blends into the sides. Or it can be a very fine fringe of bangs. But don't let anyone sell you on heavy, straight-falling bangs! They'll only make your square face look like a box.

4. Curve hair under at the bottom. It will narrow the width of the jaw. Hair curved up gives the face a wider look.

5. Hair length is best when it's below the chin line, because it will cut down on the squareness of the jaw and give you a softer look.

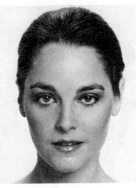

1. Make a low side part and wear a sweep of hair brushed diagonally across the forehead, held with a barrette, clip, or comb ornament. The look of more volume on one side plus the asymmetric sweep of hair will minimize the length of the face and make your head look wider.

2. Try straight-falling bangs cut to the eyebrow line. It's the classic length-cutter. Also, bangs should blend together with the sides of your hair to help shorten the overall length of your face.

3. Sides can be cut up at an angle in front; angled up to the corners of the mouth if the chin is pointy; up to the nose if not. This creates more width and less length.

4. Hair length is best when it's above the chin line because it will cut down on the length of the face.

Not part of my basic cut but a good bet for long, narrow faces is curly hair. The extra volume is very becoming, so long as you feel comfortable with curly locks, and they suit your personality.

2 The Long and Narrow Face.

This face shape is usually squeezed and compacted together, with eyes closely spaced and a chin that tends to look pointed (even if it's square). The following tips will help cut down on the length of the face and create an illusion of width. Again, if you want to stay with that 'elongated' look, skip the suggestions.

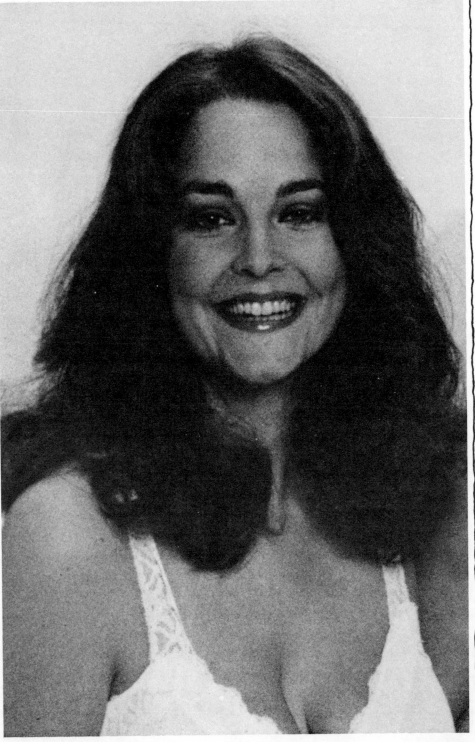

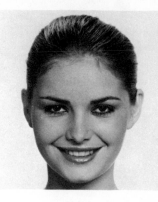

3 The Round Face.

This face shape is characterized by a lack of angular definition, with everything blending together to form a circle. The tips that follow are designed both to lengthen the face and to narrow the features. Some will even create a triangular illusion, making rounder features seem sharper. Once again, if you love your round face, stay with it!

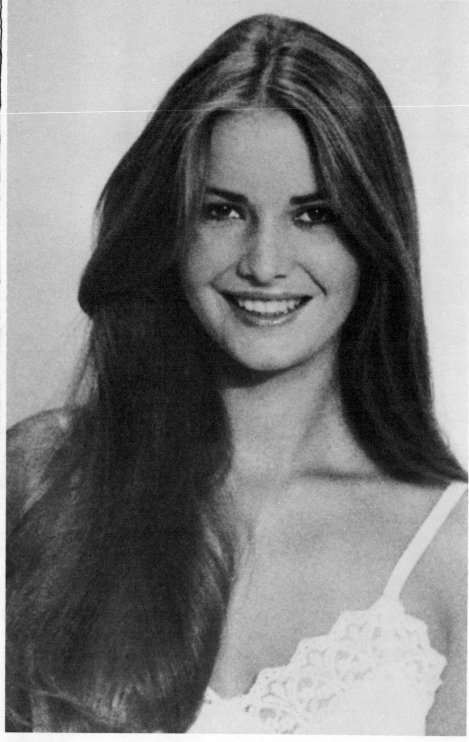

1. Try a center part. It's the most lengthening of all. But be sure your hair length is below the chin line.

2. If your hair length is above the chin line, an off-center part minimizes roundness.

3. Wear ends turned up on one side and turned under on the other. This asymmetry breaks up the roundness.

4. A bare forehead tends to lengthen the face, while bangs are a shortener. But if you insist on bangs, try curlier, fluffier side bangs and not flat, straight-falling ones.

5. Keep hair brushed away from the face. This is especially true for short angled hair. This creates extra volume and makes the face seem more triangular than round. It also narrows the width of the features.

6. The best hair length for you is 1½" below the chin line, if hair is all one length, and if the sides are cut up at an angle toward the jaw. This makes the face look longer.

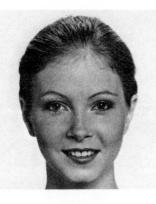

4 **The Heart-shaped or Triangular Face.** The classic heart-shaped face is characterized by a broad brow, wide cheeks, and narrow chin. The triangular face has a wide chin and narrow brow. The following tips can maximize the best and minimize the worst of either:

1. For the heart shape, try a side part with three-quarter bangs that cover one corner of your forehead. This will pare down the excessive width at the forehead and cheeks.

2. For the heart shape, wear some fullness at the bottom, with the hair coming forward onto the cheeks. This will make the chin seem wider.

3. For the heart shape, the best hair length is between the mouth and the chin line, cut evenly all around so it will soften the chin area.

4. For the classic triangular shape, the best hair length is to the chin line or below. But be sure there is fullness at the sides to balance the shape of your head. This can be done by angle-cutting: the hair on top of the head is the shortest, the hair on the sides is cut at an angle to the head, getting longer as you near the chin. Brush the hair away from the face and up toward the ear. The hair level with the top of your ear should cover the ear and then be brushed toward the chin.

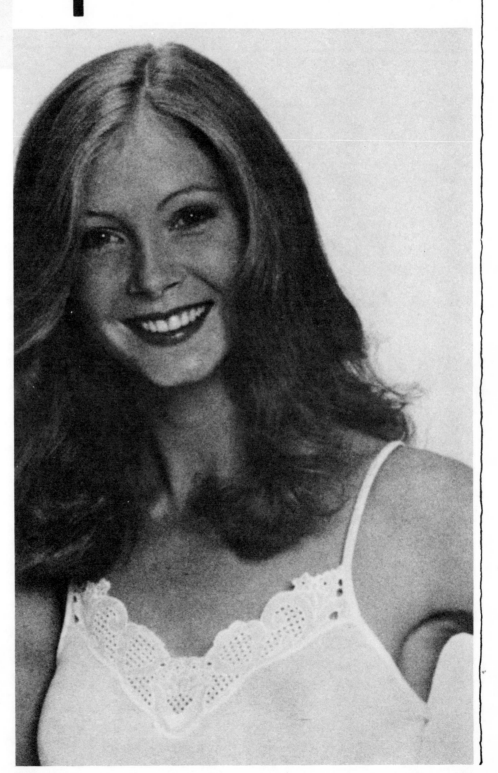

5

The Oval Face. The oval face is the most versatile—there is almost no style or cut that doesn't look sensational on it, providing you have good basic features and proportioned neck length. I do, however, have a few favorite looks for oval faces that I feel emphasize their best qualities.

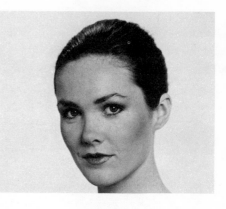

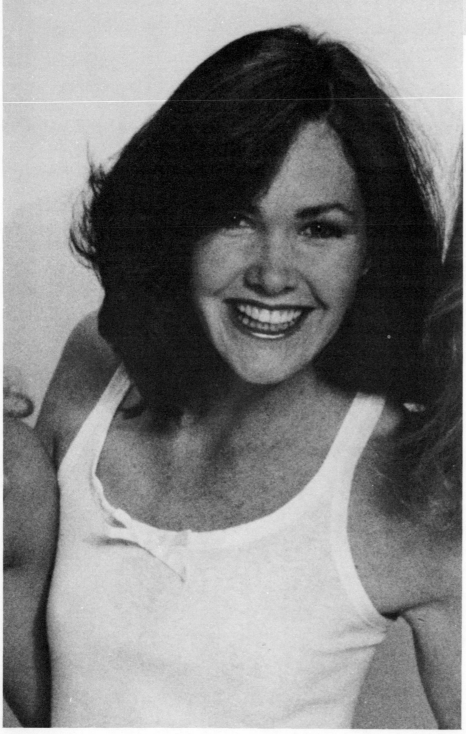

1. Try a center part or a side part with hair almost shoulder length. This is a great classic look.

2. If your hair is curly, cut it in 2½" layers starting at the top and gradually getting slightly shorter as you get down to the back of the head. The hair that rests on the nape of the neck should then be cut to the same length as that on the top (2½"). This cut will trace the shape of the head and accentuate the oval outline.

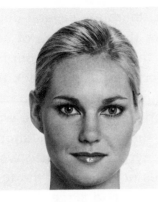

6 **The Extra-full Face.** This face shape comes close to looking like a round face, only more so. The circular shape is characterized by full cheeks and a lack of angular features. The following tips work with the fullness and stress lots of fluff and curls. Anything severe, smooth, symmetrical, or geometric should be avoided.

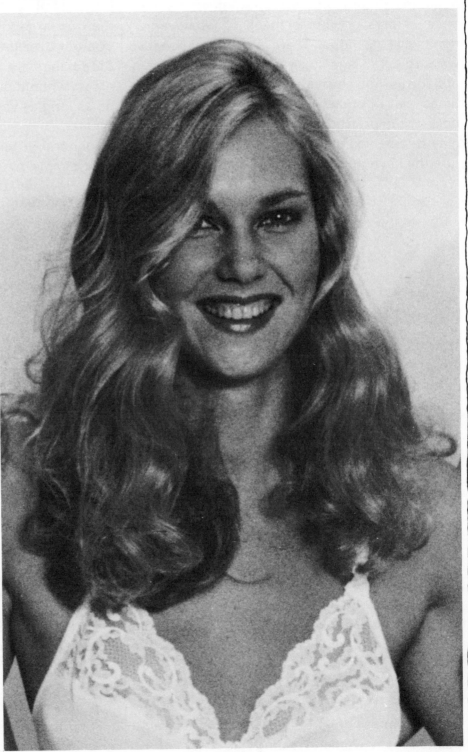

1. Both a center part and a side part have the same lengthening effect. Let your hairline guide you as to where it should be parted. (For the correct way to find your natural part, check Chapter 11.) If you use a center part, be sure the hair length is at least 2" below the chin to offset the extra roundness of the face. If you use a side part—which will also help minimize roundness—hair length should be no less than 2" below the chin.

2. As with a round face, an asymmetrical look is best. Try wearing ends turned up on one side and under on the other.

3. Try to keep hair brushed away from the face. This is especially true for short to medium-length angled hair. This creates extra volume and makes the face seem more triangular than round. It also narrows features.

4. The best hair length is not less than 2" below the chin line, if hair is all one length and if the sides are cut up at an angle toward the jaw. This will elongate the face shape.

SPECIAL FEATURES

Sometimes it's not the shape of your face that creates the problem, but a feature that somehow decided to take its own direction and not blend with the rest of the picture, so to speak. So when it comes to problem areas, whether it's your nose or ears or chin or neck or whatever . . . don't give up hope. There are lots of creative ways to cope. Again, I want to repeat that camouflage is not always the right answer. Sometimes that approach only accentuates the long nose or the protruding ears; sometimes, too, you may decide you'd rather make that special feature the keynote of your look.

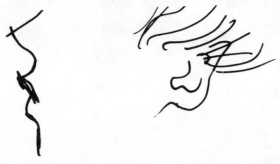

If Your Ears Stick Out, they're going to do it more through a layered cut, especially if you have fine hair. So always choose an ear-covering length or brush down just enough hair to cover the tops of your ears.

If Your Nose Is Prominent, try to avoid a center part. It acts like an arrow pointing directly at that feature. Also stay away from straight, heavy bangs. They'll only accentuate the size and shape of your nose. However, wispy side bangs or even fringe bangs will do just the opposite. Finally, avoid shorter hair.

If You Have a Problem Hairline (and by that I mean it is ragged, receding, too thin, or uneven), regular bangs aren't the only answer. Even more attractive are "baby bangs," little wisps of hair that are pulled forward on the forehead. The French Impressionist Renoir loved the look and painted many women wearing this style.

If You Wear Glasses, there are several points to be aware of. Be sure the sidepieces of your frames are not so thick that they cause your hair to stand away from your head. Next, check that your hair is long enough to wear over the ears, unless your hair is short and curly. If you wear straight-falling bangs, they should be shorter than usual (above the eyebrow) so they won't pop out over the glasses or hang over the tops. Side bangs are a good bet, and since they look nicest when they're just brushed aside, they can be as long as you like.

In general, if you wear glasses, hair should be kept simple so as not to overpower the whole face. However, there are a few exceptions.

The longer the hair, the larger your glasses should be.

A pronounced nose, other strong features, or even a wide face will look better with bigger glasses. They act as an instant distraction.

Don't hide glasses! Turn them into an asset. If you can handle them, let them be dramatic and large.

Finally, if you change your hairstyle, remember that you may have to change the style of your glasses. They should work together not only with your face but with your hair, your total image.

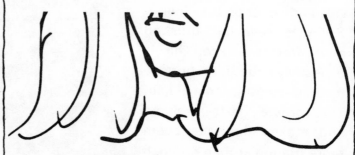

If You Have a Small or Receding Chin, the trick is to create fullness at the bottom of the face. Therefore, you'll want a cut that's all the same length and comes to about 1/2" below the chin. If you're going to have a layered cut, try making it curly and long enough so there's fullness around the chin.

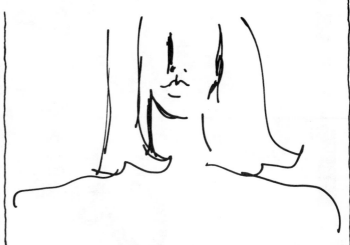

If Your Forehead Is Too Large, bangs are the traditional solution. But they don't have to have a traditional look. For example, if you have a broad, high forehead, try bangs that are heavier at the sides, wispy in the center. These will cover the forehead corners and cut the size of the forehead.

If Your Forehead Is Narrow, an off-center part is your best choice, provided your hairline is good. If it isn't, bangs can work very well (side bangs or wispy or straight-falling ones). But once again, let me repeat that sometimes a camouflage only flags the problem. Using improperly styled or cut bangs to cover up can be a disaster. So take special care in this area.

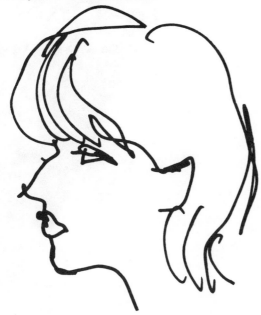

If Your Neck Is Short and Thin, you can create a charming and delicate effect by having hair cut close to the nape in back and then rounding off the corners.

If Your Neck Is Short and Thickish, hair cut longer and slightly tapered to a point in back will add an illusion of slimness and length.

If You're Big-boned and Tall, you need hair with more volume for balance. If it's too short or too flat, you'll wind up with a pinhead look.

If Your Shoulders Are Wide, shoulder-length hair will make them seem narrower.

I hope I've armed you with enough information at this point so you won't ever feel trapped by your features and face shape again. Remember, you *can* alter, change, reemphasize, or de-emphasize what you've got. This means you're free of rules and myths. Free to be you. If you're an older woman, don't feel you always have to wear a very short, layered haircut. A newer, more contemporary look is to cut hair all one length, close to the neckline in back and angled in front for softness.

If you like really long hair, don't even think about your face shape, features, or proportions. Once hair passes shoulder length, you cannot balance features any more and long hair becomes a look by itself. So if you love long hair for whatever it symbolizes for you, forget about being able to handle feature problems. Long hair tends to overpower everything else, but if it's thick, lustrous, and healthy, it's a definite plus. If that's what you want and that's how you see yourself . . . wear it!

What it all adds up to is this: Look your best with what you've got—not necessarily as it was given to you by nature, but as it can be. When you take the time to really look at yourself, feature by feature, you'll see the wonderful ways a face can be.

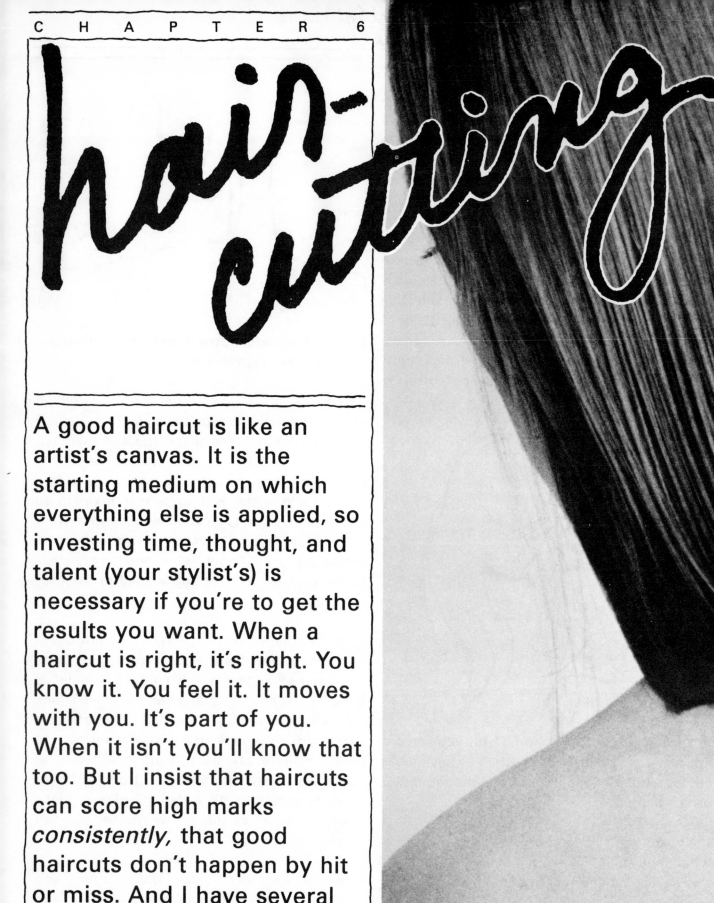

hair-cutting

A good haircut is like an artist's canvas. It is the starting medium on which everything else is applied, so investing time, thought, and talent (your stylist's) is necessary if you're to get the results you want. When a haircut is right, it's right. You know it. You feel it. It moves with you. It's part of you. When it isn't you'll know that too. But I insist that haircuts can score high marks *consistently,* that good haircuts don't happen by hit or miss. And I have several rules of thumb to guarantee clients the results they want.

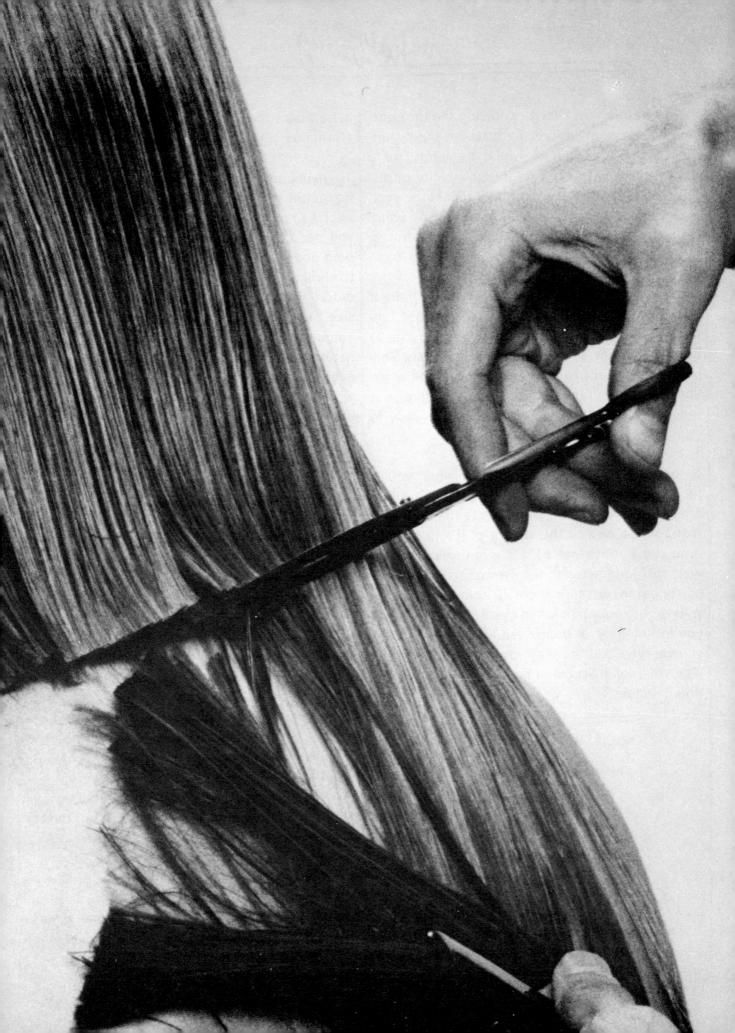

Know What You Want. Knowing the look and length you want before the scissors start snipping away is always the best beginning to a happy ending. This avoids the possibility of disappointment after the cutting process is over. However, if you're not sure about what you want, discuss it with your stylist beforehand—not in midstream (see Chapter 4).

Avoid the "One-way Cut" Trap. A haircut should not be done to achieve just one look, unless you absolutely insist on it. It's much better to have a cut that will move in any direction. This gives you the option of changing your look when you change your mood. A good haircut, like your life, should be flexible and versatile ... ready to adapt to any situation.

Know When to Cut. You'll know when you're ready for a cut better than anyone else. Suddenly your hair will become difficult to manage or it won't move well or the weight of it will start to drag the bounce out of it. It's important not to wait too long after these symptoms appear or you'll begin to think there is something really wrong with your hair when there isn't. And when you're unhappy or depressed about your hair, it shows—you feel the way you look and look the way you feel. It you're in doubt, consult my "cutting calendar":

Short hair
(layered) . . . . . every six weeks
Above-shoulder hair
(all one length or angled)
. . . . . every eight to ten weeks
At-shoulder hair
(all one length or angled)
. . . . . every ten to twelve weeks.

A few situations can accelerate this timetable. Warm climates, for instance, cause hair to grow much faster. Also, a fever or anything else that generates excessive body heat—such as regular strenuous exercise—will speed up growth.

There is one other time when a haircut is in order no matter what length you have, and that's when your hair starts to split at the ends. Then what you need is a "health cut," which involves snipping no more than a ¼" all around—just enough to eliminate the split ends. If you ignore this condition, the split ends will eventually cause extensive damage. And because they reduce the amount of oxygen that penetrates the shaft, the natural rate of hair growth will slow down. However, once split ends are gone your growth rate will return to normal. So make sure you treat them when they appear.

Singeing hair as a way of combatting split ends is a method that started in the barber shops many years ago; it is still done, even in some women's salons. Burning the hair does destroy split ends; however, the new ones that you're left with are more damaged than the original ones. Therefore, the results are short, more noticeable split ends. My advice: Don't ever singe.

Don't Be Bullied. One thing to remember about haircutting is not to be bullied by a scissor-happy stylist or by one who doesn't listen to what you want. If you ask for a 1" trim, then that's what you should get. Be firm. *You're* the boss. It's impossible to stop once the cutting process has begun, so be very, very specific about how much you want to be cut or trimmed. If a particular stylist has the reputation of always cutting too much, you should find this out during the communications meeting ... not after.

Don't Be Misled. There are a few helpful hints you should know so you won't be misled during the cutting process. When asking for a classic cut, chin or shoulder length, be aware that straight hair is shorter when dry than when wet. On the other hand, curly hair looks shorter wet and longer after it has been blow-dried because the pulling action of the brush will straighten the curls. If you let curly hair dry naturally, it'll look shorter. So don't be duped into thinking that the stylist has missed the cutting mark until you see the results dry.

Think Seasonal. Winter and summer months change our life-styles and along with that the way we dress, what we do, and how much time we have to do it in. Long hair for summer has become fairly traditional for many women because they can do more with it: pin it up at the beach, tie it back playing tennis, wear it down on an ordinary evening, or up for flair on special evenings. So think about that before you decide to have your hair cut short in June. Conversely, shorter hair for winter is more a fashion convenience than a weather consideration. These are months when women like to keep their hair away from turtlenecks, cowls, scarves, and high collars. Shorter hair also means shorter caring time, so think about that bonus when your work schedule begins to fill in and you find yourself canceling hair appointments at the beauty salon.

KINDS OF CUTS

There are four ways to cut hair: razor/taper, layered, angled, blunt. Certain cuts are better than others for certain kinds of hair. Let's discuss these in greater detail.

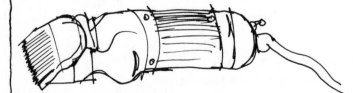

Razor or Taper Cuts. Using a sharp razor instead of cutting scissors was a very popular procedure decades ago. And it was a major cause of split ends because the razor cut left hair ends so thin that they split almost instantly. My advice is to stay away from any stylist who favors razors.

Layered and Angled Cuts. These are probably the most common and popular haircuts today. However, they're not for everyone. I'd like to give you a few guidelines about what type hair should or should not be cut in these ways.

Straight fine hair should never be cut in layers. This only removes the precious little bulk you need all over your head. Unfortunately, a lot of women think the opposite is true. Once straight fine hair is cut in layers, the only way it can have fullness is by teasing and spraying—two unhealthy and certainly out-of-date procedures. There is only one exception to this rule, and that's when straight fine hair has had a body wave. This gives the illusion of thicker hair and will make the finer strands seem fuller and bouncier, so a layered cut will work properly then. The very best and most natural way for straight fine hair to be cut is the same length all around or at an angle in the front for softness and manageability. How short or long you go depends on your features and shape of face.

Wavy or curly fine hair (whether naturally curly or permed) can be cut in layers or angled, especially if you're after height and fullness. This will also give you the chance to use your own curl or wave to create a natural look—one free of work and totally free in movement.

Blunt Cuts. Hair is cut the same length all around, with no layering or tapering.

Thick, curly, or straight hair looks well with a blunt cut, which gives fullness. That's the beauty of it. This cut also makes hair easy to control, no matter what length.

55

TEN CLASSIC HAIRCUTS

By "classic" I mean a look that will never go out of style. A look that's not a fad or passing fancy. Because of this, a "classic" is one of the easiest looks to have and to keep. The variations on these ten themes are endless, but they are the building blocks for all other looks—and one of them will probably fit your face.

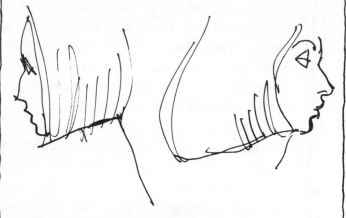

1. Hair all one length, shorter in back and slightly longer in front. It may be worn from chin length to as long as you like.

2. Hair all one length, slightly longer in back and angled slightly or sharply up in front. The angle cut may be done from chin length to about 2" below the shoulder. Longer hair doesn't really look well with this kind of cut.

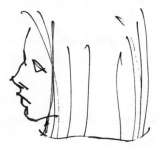

3. Hair all one length and even all around. This is a very classic look, the length depending on what's best for your features and face shape. This cut is very good starting 2" below chin level, but it could go longer or shorter.

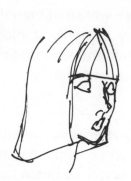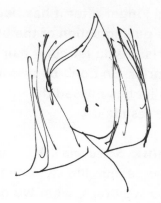

4. Hair all one length with straight-falling bangs. Hair may be angled up toward the front and longer in back; short in back and slightly longer in front; or simply straight and even all around. If bangs are worn, hair length should ideally be above the shoulder. When it's longer than that, you develop a "little girl" look. (Of course, if that's what you want, let it grow!)

5. Hair all one length with side bangs. Any length hair is good, again depending on your features and the look you're after. I particularly like side bangs with hair cut the same length all around or cut up at an angle.

6. Shorter hair all one length. This cut is angled up in the front to give a tapered look in back, and the back shaped close to the neck. The front and top areas should be one length and very smooth. It can be worn with sides and back smooth and straight down or with sides brushed away from the face to blend in with the back. The best length is above the chin.

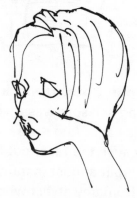

7. Curly, wavy, or permed hair. May be cut very short or go as long as above the shoulder. Hair is cut in layers all over. The sides and back may be as long as you like, but it's best if the crown and front are no more than 3″ long so that those sections don't collapse and lie flat after blow-drying or setting.

8. Very short hair that's straight or wavy. Hair is cut in layers about 1½″ long all over to give a very cropped effect.

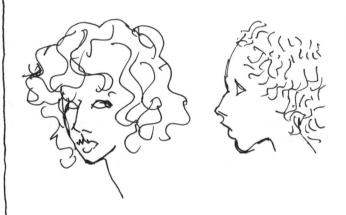

9. Long, wavy hair. For hair worn at shoulder length or slightly longer, this is the preferred cut for curly hair or hair with a strong natural wave. Hair is cut in a long angle all over and dried. The crown and front should be cut shorter than the rest so they fluff properly when dry.

10. Hair ½″ or ¼″ below the ear. Hair should be angled about ½″ to 1″ all around the head. Be sure the back is nape length or longer. Or keep it blunt-cut all over.

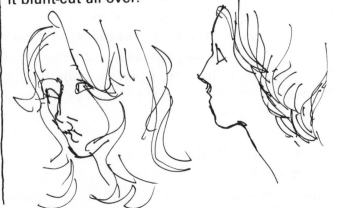

TIPS ON HAIRCUTS

Start at Eye Level. I believe a stylist must see your overall appearance before he or she starts cutting. I always have my clients stand up in front of a full-length mirror, since I can never get the right perspective of their bodies and features if they are lower than my eye level or sitting in a chair. Think about it. When a tailor is marking a skirt for hemming, doesn't he ask you to stand straight and tall? In this position too, a stylist can best evaluate the length of your neck, width of your shoulders, your overall body impression. He can then suggest a length and look most appropriate for your height and proportions.

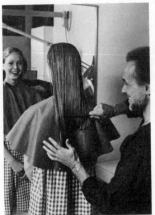

Where to Part Is Important. One sure way of creating a flexible haircut is to be sure your stylist starts with either a precise center part or none at all. Never begin with an off-center part. This only results in more long hairs on one side and short ones on the other. What you get, in effect, is a lopsided haircut.

Cut Hair Wet. If someone approaches you with scissors when your hair is dry, run to the nearest water source or else expect disastrous results. Why? Simply because you cannot *see* the natural direction of the wave when your hair is dry. It might be disguised from the blow-drying or setting you did in the morning. When hair is wet, the stylist can clearly determine its direction. There is one exception to my "cut when wet" rule, and it applies to short, frizzy hair. It is easier for a stylist to see growth, direction, and movement with this type of hair when it is dry. However, I advise that frizzy hair be shampooed and conditioned immediately after the cut, and that the stylist recheck the cut while the hair is wet to be sure of perfect results.

If You Want One Length, Think "Duplex." This refers to a two-level not a two-layered look. Short or long hair of one length should be "duplexed"—that is, cut with the back a bit shorter than the front. Why? First, hair in the back grows twice as fast as sides and front, and if your hair is the same length in front as it is in back, in a few months you'll find yourself with a necktail and everything will be out of proportion. Second, when hair is cut shorter in the back, it will swing forward with you when you walk as the weight of the longer hair comes forward. And the "duplex" is great if you wear hair swept behind your ears. Leaving the back shorter than the sides makes the sides look even with the back when they're worn behind the ears.

BANGS

Unfortunately, bangs do not compliment every face. The proper hairline, hair texture, and face shape are all necessary for perfect bangs. So make sure you've got some positives going for you before the first snip. Otherwise, the mistake may take nine to twelve months to grow out.

What to watch for:

Widow's peaks and cowlicks make bangs a near impossibility because bangs must lie flat on the forehead with no protrusions or separations. A widow's peak is a triangular swatch of hair that lies on your forehead in the middle of your hairline. That hair grows up and back and will never lie flat unless it is forced against its natural direction. The same is true of cowlicks. Found almost anywhere around the head, cowlicks are sections of hair that will not lie flat. If you happen to have a cowlick near the front hairline, bangs will be a nusiance. You could blow dry or set them,

but they probably won't stay that way for long. If you have a widow's peak and can't live without bangs, keep them long (to the tip of your nose) and use a blow-dryer or roller to close the split. Or work with the split and blow the bangs back toward the sides. The second method will hold longer than the first. But whatever method you use, know that you're forcing the hair against its growth—something I don't recommend.

Texture and Quality. Both are important for great-looking bangs:

If your bangs are curly or wavy, you're one of the lucky ones, especially if they curl properly and are cut a bit longer than straight bangs. Otherwise, the curl can be controlled by a roller or blow-dyer. Extreme cases of frizziness will look better straightened. Try a mild relaxing solution, which can cause minimal damage but will create just the look you may be after. (Remember, however that in humid weather it's difficult to keep curly bangs manageable; unless you're willing to invest the time and energy to keep them looking right, skip bangs.)

If your hair is straight, your bangs can be permed for a curlier look. This is also a painless way to let bangs grow out. Wavy bangs add great flare to an otherwise dull, straight look.

If your hair is fine, avoid short pieces around the hairline. These only remove whatever little bulk you may have. It's better to keep hair all one length around your face. Don't opt for straight-falling bangs for the same reason. If you can't live without them, be sure they are not cut behind the temple hairline. I prefer "baby bangs" for people with this type of fine hair or for those with bad hairlines.

Baby Bangs. Whatever is the cause of your not-so-good hairline (broken hair around hairline; irregular hairline; receding hairline), don't hide it—

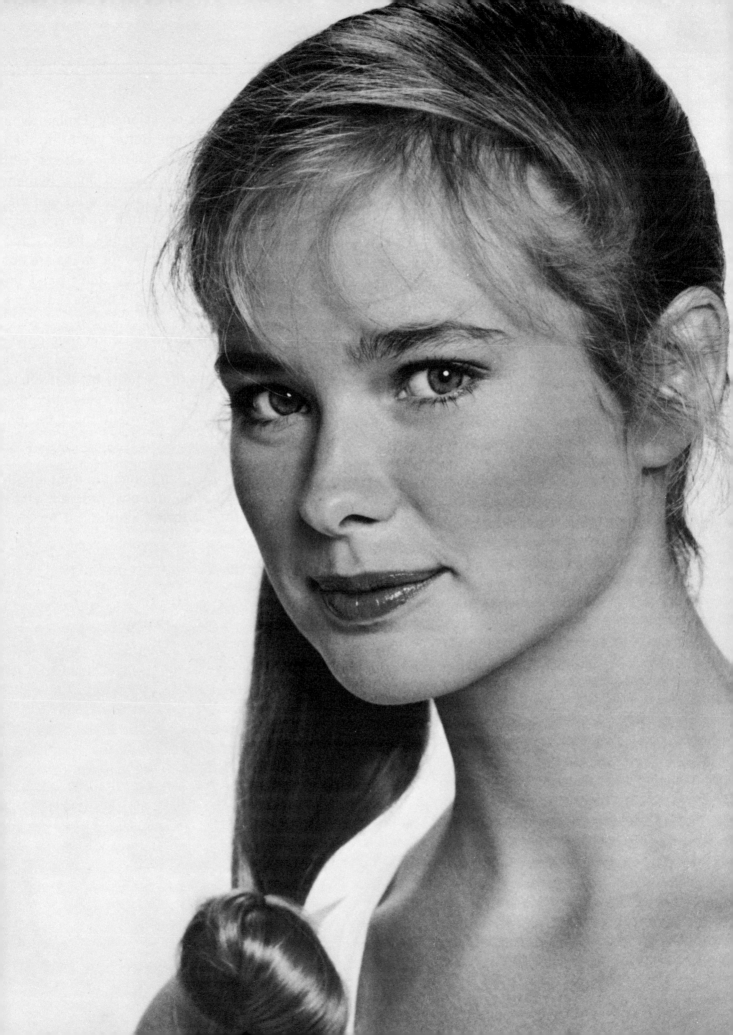

play with it, make the most of it. Use the little pieces of hair you already have around the hairline, and if there aren't enough (which there probably won't be), take some from just behind the hairline at the top and sides of your head. Pull or brush these pieces forward toward your face. This will instantly create a fuller look. And you'll be amazed at what an interesting and stylish hairline you can effect without much effort.

Two-way Bangs. Yes, there are bangs that can switch into nonbangs and then back into bangs when you want them. They are supercasual and side-swept and should be cut no shorter than midway up the bridge of your nose. Then simply brush them to the side, and what you create is a whimsical, wispy look.

Bangs and Glasses. If you wear glasses, tell the stylist before he or she makes the first cut. And go into detail. Indicate whether you wear them all the time or occasionally. Explain what shape and style they are. Better yet, bring them with you. Modern, simple frames look better with bangs than heavy, old-fashioned ones. Remember, bangs and glasses are accessories and they must work together. Very often when you get a new haircut, it'll be time for new frames, too. From a practical point, side-swept bangs are better with glasses because they don't need the constant trimming that straight bangs require.

Bangs as a Camouflage. Don't overpower your face with heavy bangs. Some women hide behind them. If that's the security blanket you've chosen for yourself, okay. But remember that bangs really should compliment the face, not camouflage it.

Do It Yourself. Keeping bangs the right length can become a big time and cost problem, since it's impractical to go to the hairdresser for con-

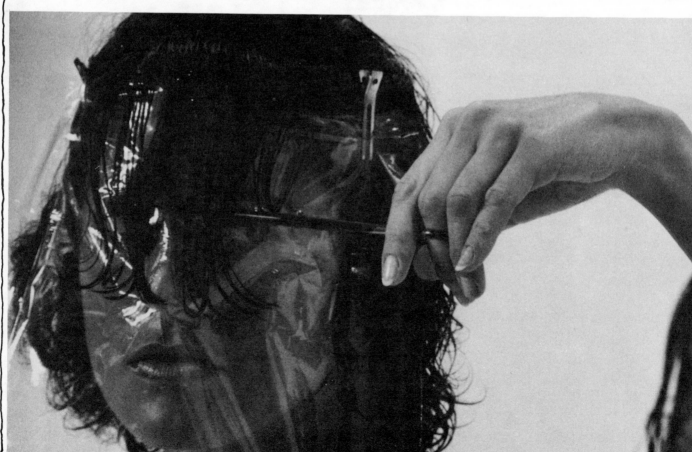

stant trimming. Once in a while a stylist won't mind a few free snips. But if you need help every two weeks, it will be costly. So why not learn how to trim bangs yourself? It's not very difficult if you know the basics. Here's how it's done.

1. Bangs should extend not more than 1" to 2½" below the hairline and should be cut from a point on the very top of the head. This is the tip of the triangle.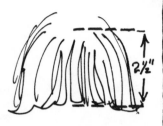
2. The sides of the triangle are formed by cutting the sides diagonally.
3. Don't start bangs from the very top of the head unless the overall length of the hair is bang-length. Straight, full bangs should reach the bottom of the eyebrow. Straight side bangs should stop at the bridge of your nose. And curly side bangs should stop at the tip of your nose.

A few tips. Don't cut too far into the side hairline. This widens the bangs too much and removes the length needed at the sides. The result is that the hair begins to look finer than it is. Don't cut too much from the top either. This thickens the bangs, will make you feel top-heavy, and creates a look that is out of proportion with the rest of your head (unless the hair is cut to bang-length all over)

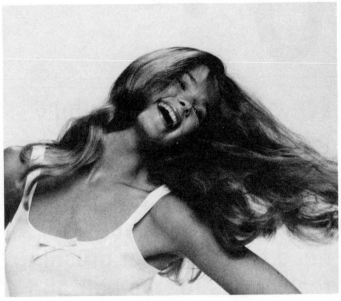

THE TEST OF A GOOD CUT

When your newly cut hair has been dried, try my **shake-out** test. First, shake your head from side to side with vigor. Then bend over at the waist, letting the hair hang down. Shake a few more times. Straighten up and do a few more finishing shakes. If your hair falls into its natural line after all this, you've had a great cut.

I hope now that you understand the importance of a good haircut and that getting what you want is not just a hit-or-miss propositon, but entirely possible—especially if you keep everything you've just read in mind. If you truly want the very best look for your hair, put in extra time and effort at the haircutting stage. Beause the cut is the key to everything that follows.

brushing

Why is it that we faithfully brush our cats and dogs to give them shiny, healthy coats and then forget about our own hair? Maybe we need to learn what brushing really does for the hair and whether the old "hundred strokes a night" formula is fact or fiction.

The benefits of brushing are certainly real, and very important. Brushing is one of the best and easiest ways to guarantee yourself beautiful hair. It stimulates the scalp, increases circulation, distributes oils, and adds fullness and shine to the

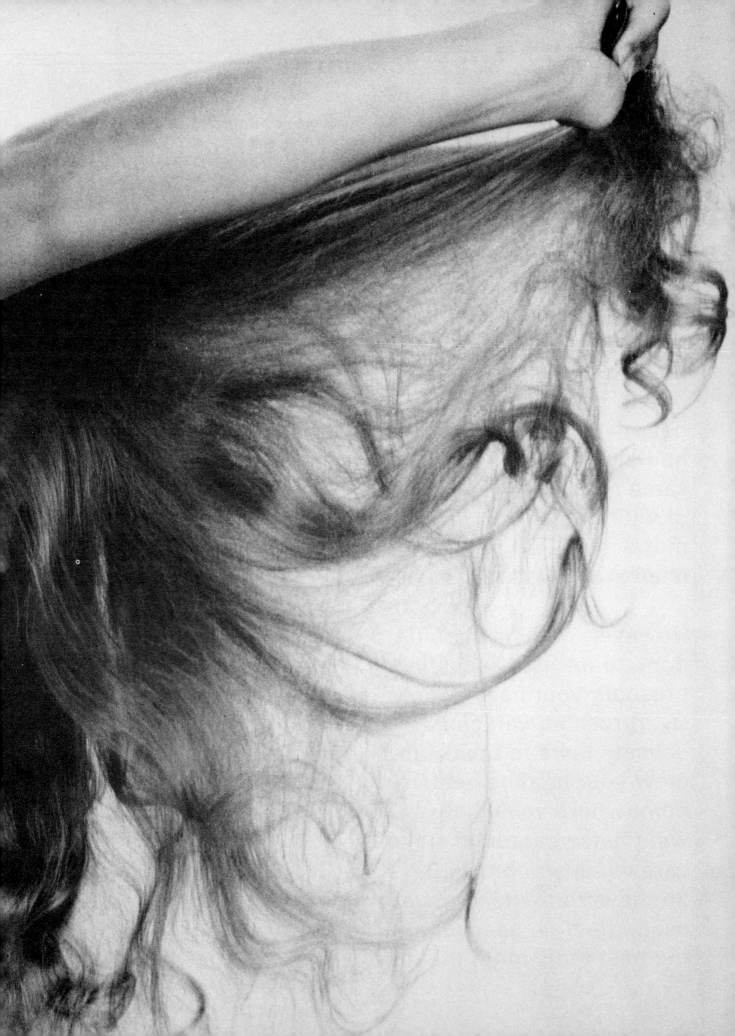

hair. You needn't adhere strictly to the hundred strokes regimen, but a certain amount of time spent brushing guarantees that each hair follicle will absorb sufficient oxygen and nutrients to maintain its health. After all, consider how much taking a deep breath helps you to feel better—why not give your hair a chance to have that same healthy feeling? Think of your hair as you do the muscles in your body. Both need exercise to stay in shape.

However, nothing should be done to excess—including brushing your hair. Overbrushing can cause delicate hairs to break, and mow your hairline back to a point where you'll have to wear hats year-round. Take care when you brush: Be attentive to the technique used, the time needed, and the best tools to do the job.

· · · · · · · T·O·O·L·S · · · · · · · ·

Choosing the right brush should be an intelligent decision and not a spur-of-the-moment one. This can only happen when you have the correct product information at your fingertips. It can get pretty confusing to sort out what's best for you, because there are scores of different shapes and sizes on the market, and because selecting the right style for you depends on several things: the texture of your hair, the sensitivity of your scalp, the condition of your budget. For general use, look for a brush with a rounded or semicylindrical shape and rounded bristles that are not uniform in length. These give a better performance than blunt-cut bristles because their contoured shape will follow the natural contour of your

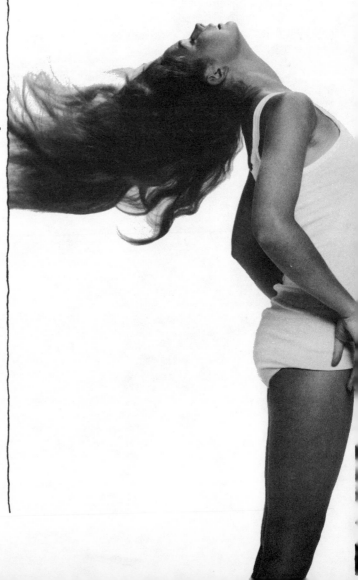

head. After all, your head isn't flat, so why should your head be? And bristles that are cut off straight will be sharp, with a tendency to irritate the scalp and pull the hair, ultimately causing breakage and split ends.

There are as many different types of bristle as there are styles of brush, and which type you use will depend on your hair. At one time natural bristle was recommended as the "only and best" for hairbrushing. But with modern formulations, many of today's synthetic bristles are also very effective. This gives the consumer many more options when selecting a brush. Remember, though, that different bristles do different things for your hair.

Natural Bristle. The most expensive of all bristle types. It is usually (but not always) constructed with a cushiony rubber base. This rubber cushion reduces 75 to 85 percent of the static electricity generated during brushing and also eliminates hair breakage because the pliable rubber base tends to give, not tug, with each stroke. Soft natural bristle is good for very fine hair or treated hair (which tends to break very easily). Hard natural bristle (boar) is good for any texture, including treated hair. And it will outlast nylon.

Mixed Bristle. Usually a combination of natural bristle and nylon. Good for any texture hair except fine. Excellent for thin hair, but not recommended for sensitive scalps. Mixed bristle is less expensive than natural bristle.

Nylon Bristle. Good for any texture hair, but not for sensitive scalps. Also good for wet hair comb-outs. Generally inexpensive. Today's technology produces nylon bristles that can be very close to natural bristles in performance. One of the most effective is the "hi-lo" nylon bristle that is tapered and smooth at the end.

Plastic Bristle. Usually constructed on a rubber base. The best known brand is Denman, available with 7 rows of bristle (9 rows become too bulky). Excellent because it untangles wet or dry hair without pulling. Fits comfortably in the hand for styling ease. Highly recommended for blow-drying, especially the new wash-and-wear cuts, because it gives a smoother look. Easy to clean because bristles are set in a detachable rubber base.

· · · · · T·E·C·H·N·I·Q·U·E · · · · ·

There is a proper way to brush your hair—and it's *not* the old-fashioned method of starting from the front and stroking toward the back! If you brush your hair that way, you can wreck your hairline and reduce the crown of your head to stubble, because these are the weakest parts of your hair.

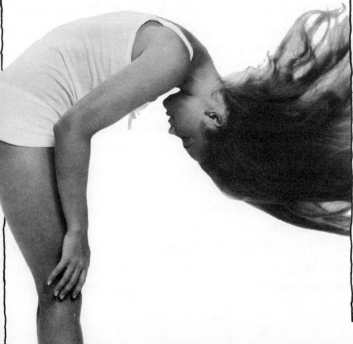

Here is the best brushing system to use:

1. Bend forward at the waist. Hold the head down and brush away from the scalp, starting at the neckline and working your way toward the front. This will cut down on the brushstrokes around your hairline and crown, and help prevent the breakage of the delicate hairs in these areas. Furthermore, this method of brushing—with your head down—helps promote circulation of blood to the scalp.

2. Flip your hair back to normal position.

3. Repeat the process again if you have the time.

When you've given your hair a thorough brushing, try aerating it with the styling method I call **natural teasing**. It gives fullness to your hair and gives your body a limbering and energizing stretch at the same time:

1. Bend forward at the waist, letting your hair hang down freely.

2. Now come up to a straight position, flinging your hair and head back.

3. Repeat the exercise five times and on the last round before you come up, shake your head from side to side.

4. Stand up, pat a few hairs in place, and you have instant body.

Whether your hair is long or short, shaking makes it stand up from the scalp—without teasing. Teasing is extremely damaging because it breaks hair and causes split ends. It not only creates an unattractive and old-fashioned wiglike look, but requires the use of hair spray (another hair and lung enemy) to keep flyaway strands in place. My advice: Avoid teasing at all costs and try my natural method instead if you want your hair to look active, alive, and free.

Timing. When—and for how long—should you brush your hair? Anytime is a good time, but there are special slots in the day that will work best. Brush every morning. This wakes up your scalp. Brush before shampooing. This is a must.

Make sure you use vigorous strokes in every direction to free hair of tangles or knots (see Chapter 8). If you set your hair, brush after setting—brush it in all directions and then shake your head around. This will smooth out any lines or ridges left by rollers, curling irons, or clips. Brush every evening. Never go to sleep with pins, rubber bands, or even curls still in place. Your hair should be free and relaxed, just as you should be for a good night's rest.

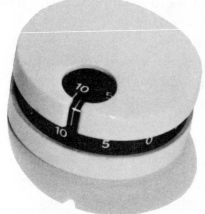

Timing tip: Instead of counting strokes, try using a 3-minute egg timer. This sets a limit while it frees your mind to think, plan for the day ahead, or even meditate.

BRUSH CARE

Keeping brushes and combs clean is as important as selecting them: If you don't use clean tools, you're only adding last week's dirt and grime to freshly washed hair.

Here's the best way to care for brushes:

1. Soak for a few minutes in warm (not hot) soapy water. Use your favorite shampoo for the suds. Never leave a brush soaking overnight. This will loosen the bristles and cause the base to deteriorate.

2. Scrub gently between the rows with an old toothbrush.

3. Dry with bristles facing down so the water will drip away from the base (water accumulating around the base can also loosen the bristles).

BRUSH CHART

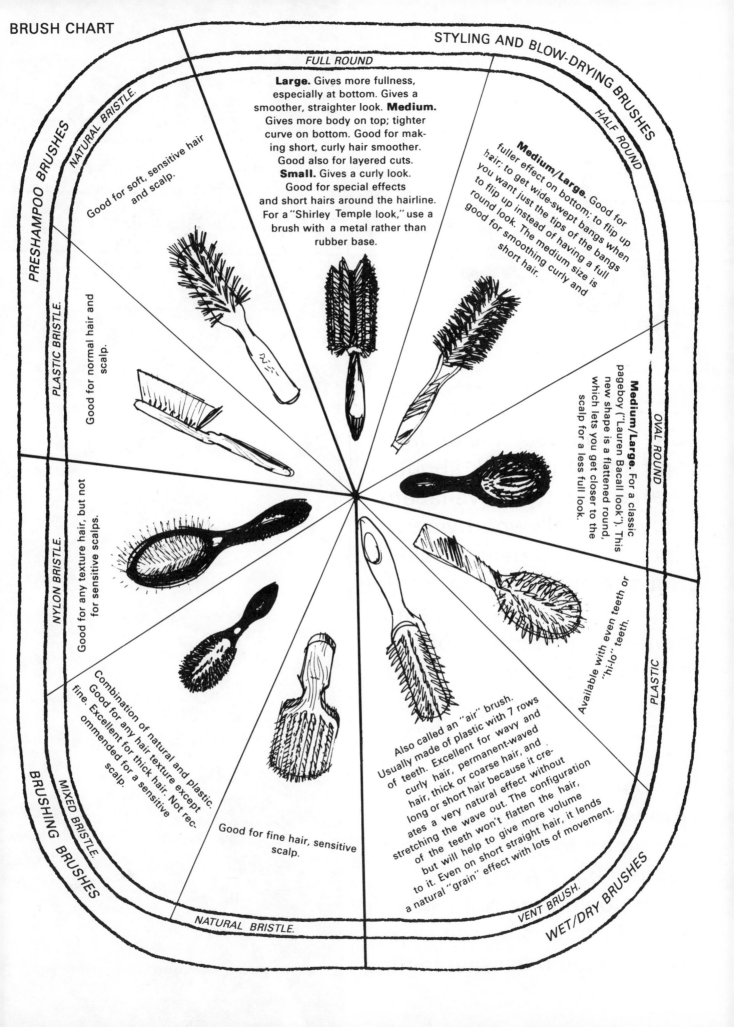

STYLING AND BLOW-DRYING BRUSHES

PRESHAMPOO BRUSHES

BRUSHING BRUSHES

WET/DRY BRUSHES

FULL ROUND

HALF ROUND

OVAL ROUND

NATURAL BRISTLE.

PLASTIC BRISTLE.

NYLON BRISTLE.

MIXED BRISTLE.

NATURAL BRISTLE.

VENT BRUSH.

PLASTIC

Good for soft, sensitive hair and scalp.

Good for normal hair and scalp.

Good for any texture hair, but not for sensitive scalps.

Combination of natural and plastic. Good for any hair texture except fine. Excellent for thick hair. Not recommended for a sensitive scalp.

Good for fine hair, sensitive scalp.

Large. Gives more fullness, especially at bottom. Gives a smoother, straighter look. **Medium.** Gives more body on top; tighter curve on bottom. Good for making short, curly hair smoother. Good also for layered cuts. **Small.** Gives a curly look. Good for special effects and short hairs around the hairline. For a "Shirley Temple look," use a brush with a metal rather than rubber base.

Medium/Large. Good for fuller effect on bottom: to flip up hair; to get wide-swept bangs when you want just the tips of the bangs to flip up instead of having a full round look. The medium size is good for smoothing curly and short hair.

Medium/Large. For a classic pageboy ("Lauren Bacall look"). This new shape is a flattened round, which lets you get closer to the scalp for a less full look.

Available with even teeth or "hi-lo" teeth.

Also called an "air" brush. Usually made of plastic with 7 rows of teeth. Excellent for wavy and curly hair, permanent-waved hair, thick or coarse hair, and long or short hair because it creates a very natural effect without stretching the wave out. The configuration of the teeth won't flatten the hair, but will help to give more volume to it. Even on short straight hair, it lends a natural "grain" effect with lots of movement.

shampoo

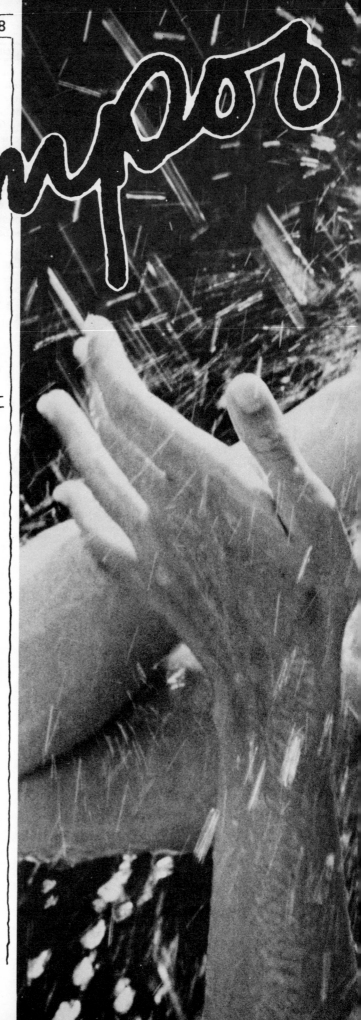

Say "shampoo" these days and lots of us think about Warren Beatty's love-laced movie, a Hollywood view of sets, sex, and beauty salons. But shampooing is really the heart of hair care. And for something we do so often—sometimes daily—we need to have the correct answers to questions such as these: Are you preparing your hair properly for shampooing? Are you using the best shampoo for your type and texture hair? Are you shampooing the right way or are you scrubbing too hard, soaping too much, detangling

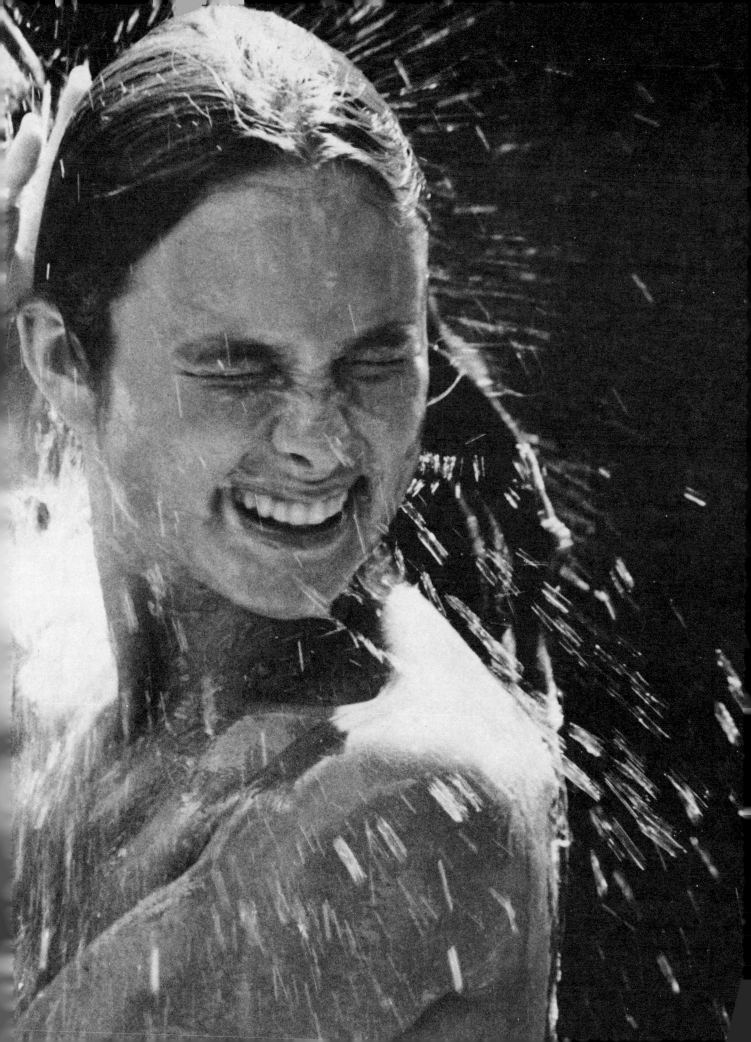

knots too roughly?

Luckily, you don't have to be a professional to learn the answers, although it's the professionals who have made shampooing the healthy, luxurious ritual it often is today. Until the mid-1930s, cake soap was about the only product available for cleansing hair. Then along came a few brand-name shampoos, special preparations specifically for cleaning the hair and scalp. These very early shampoos were simple liquid coconut-oil soap products that had an advantage over regular soap bars because they lathered quickly and thickly, rinsed more freely, and gave better results in hard water.

Since then tremendous advancements have been made in chemical formulations and technology. Most modern shampoos now contain sulfates of fatty alcohols that are derived from natural vegetable oils (olive, palm, etc.). These fatty alcohol sulfates belong to a group of products labeled *surfactants,* which give many advantages to shampoo: They are soluble in water, can be regulated as to lather and cleansing power, and facilitate film-free rinsing. Soap is almost never an ingredient in modern formulas; instead, in addition to surfactants, our shampoos contain lather stabilizers, antifermenting agents, lubricators (used especially for dry, colored, or permed hair), softeners, and often perfume to override the raw material's odor and give shampoo a pleasant fragrance.

SELECTING A SHAMPOO

With all these components in one bottle, merely choosing a shampoo may seem complicated. Just as you do when you read food labels, check the ingredients in shampoos—it will help you ascertain that you're using the best formula for your hair. Today we all want a shampoo to do more than just clean the 100,000 or so hairs on our heads. We want it to add shine, body, bounce, softness, stylability. We insist it combat dryness, dandruff, oil, dullness, and on and on. The manufacturers have responded with a host of enrichers from lanolin to protein, herbs to eggs, milk to beer, vitamins to minerals. All these additives only add to the cost and romance surrounding the "right" choice because they usually go down the drain in the rinse water.

What you should look for in a good shampoo is its ability to dissolve grime, oil, and dirt without harming the hair. When applied and lathered, a proper shampoo gathers the dulling film caused by dirt so you can rinse it away easily. I recommend you stick with a shampoo formulated with an average pH or acid balance. And since most products on the market *are* acid-balanced, there's no need to worry about making the wrong decision. The pH factor of a shampoo indicates the degree of acidity or alkalinity in the formula. A pH count in the 4 to 8.5 range tells you it is balanced and neutral. Below 4 the shampoo is more acidic, which means the hair cuticles—those tiny, overlapping scales covering the hair shaft—become resistant to cleansing. A pH of over 8.5 is quite alkaline, and over 11 will actually dissolve hair. Shampoos with no pH label rarely have an acid balance below 6, so don't worry. A pH-balanced shampoo has many benefits: It is less harsh on color-treated hair; it is an excellent cleanser; it helps keep hair shiny because it keeps the hair cuticle flat. But probably the most important reason for using a pH-balanced shampoo is for the health of your scalp. Hair loses only a minimal amount of acid during washing, but the scalp suffers much more.

Switching Shampoos Is Okay. In fact, I advise that you try not to use just one brand of shampoo. Find a few that work for you and then alternate or rotate them biweekly or monthly, so your hair keeps responding to the ingredients.

A Word of Caution. Steer clear of "conditioner" shampoos that look and feel like grease when applied. The majority of these contain heavy doses of lanolin, which simply coats the hair with oil.

Learn about Lather. Don't be misled by a shampoo that doesn't lather. A lot of us mistakenly believe that the more suds a shampoo makes, the more effectively it cleans. This is *false.* Some of the best formulas have low-sudsing action and still leave the hair squeaky clean. An important factor in lathering is the quality of the water you are washing with. Hard water, for instance, reduces sudsing and does not rinse well. If you live in a hard-water area, use a shampoo that does not contain soap. Generally speaking, most products on the market do not contain soap, but there are certain cream-type shampoos that might include some amount of soap. Also, an effective hard-water shampoo should include a chelating agent, an ingredient that works by scooping-up certain minerals in the hard water. Of course, the best solution of all is to use the best water of all. The kind you collect in the bucket . . . rainwater.

SPECIAL SHAMPOOS

Drugstore shelves are filled with formulas for problem hair and scalp. Before you decide to use any of them, be sure you diagnose your condition properly—if necessary, with the advice of your doctor—so you know you are applying the correct product.

Tar shampoos are usually prescribed for acute dandruff problems. They will loosen dead skin on the scalp, making it easier to wash away.

Dandruff shampoos containing selenium sulfide are effective for mild dandruff conditions and consistently itching scalp. Use only one soaping and follow up with an application of your own shampoo. This will return the hair to its normal acidity and also counteract the strong odor of the treatment. Remember, too, that dandruff shampoo dries out hair, so if your hair is extremely dry to begin with, stay away from these formulations. Instead, have frequent washings with a protein-enriched shampoo. Or try my dandruff-control rinse recipe (see Chapter 9).

Henna shampoos are supposed to give hair shine and body. Neutral henna coats the shafts, giving them more bulk and more body. But a word of caution is in order here. If you don't rinse the henna out well, the gritty residue can be abrasive and damaging to the hair. And if you rinse it away completely, you negate the whole purpose of applying it in the first place.

If you're looking for extra *shine,* a henna shampoo will give it to you—but only the first time you use it. Repeated applications coat the hair, and the result is dullness instead of shine. My advice is to limit henna shampooing to no more than 3 applications a year. (For more on henna, see Chapter 13.)

Dry shampoos are good for traveling, on camping trips when water is at a premium, or when the doctor has asked you to keep your head warm and dry. A few products are available that spray on and brush out dirt. They're effective as a stopgap measure, but nothing is as good as a "shower shampoo."

HOW OFTEN TO SHAMPOO

I find no truth to the warning that you should not wash your hair every day. I believe hair can be shampooed almost as often as you wash your hands—if you use the proper shampoo. If you are a daily washer, one of the easiest, fastest, and most effective ways to shampoo is in the shower. Treat yourself to a removable shower head. It's great for hard-to-reach areas; its pulsating action massages and relaxes the scalp; and its power spray does a thorough and stimulating rinsing job, especially on long hair. If you're not a shower lover and prefer to wash your hair over the sink basin, pay particular attention to the rinsing process at the neckline and across the front hairline.

Natural (untreated) hair, whether short or long, should be shampooed every day to keep it at its best. A daily regimen is even more important if you live in a city where grime and pollution seem to make hair dirtier faster. If you do shampoo every day, it's best to only use one soaping. This keeps hair from becoming too soft and flyaway.

Treated hair needs special care in shampooing because it is more porous and absorbs more shampoo. So use a very small amount and al-

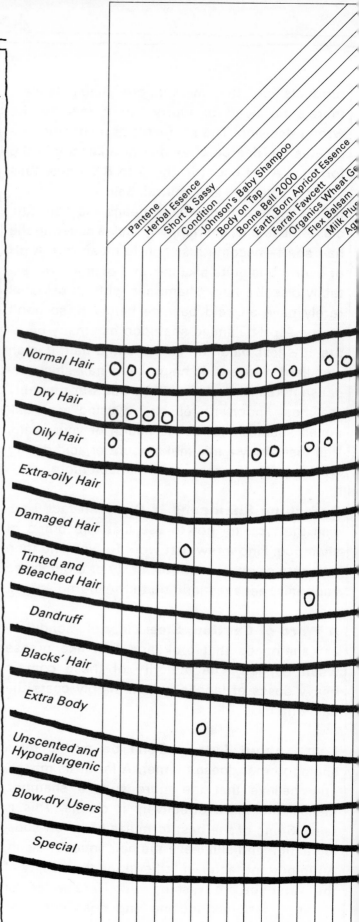

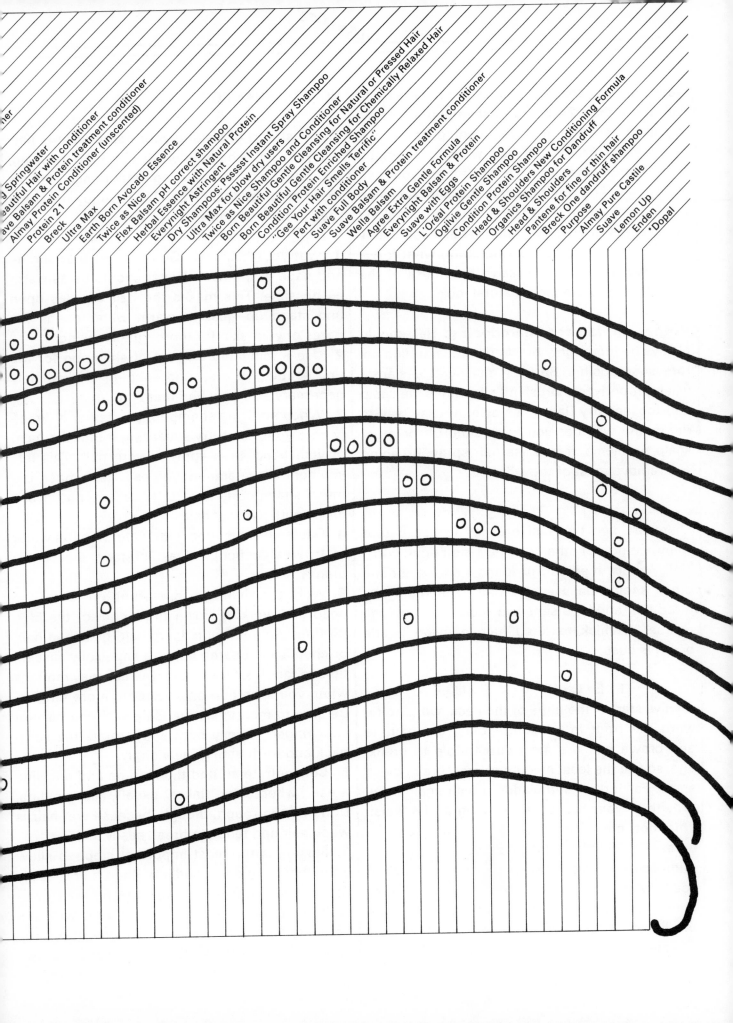

ways only one soaping. But it's not necessary to wait more than 24 hours to shampoo after having had a permanent, a straightening, or any other chemical process. If you want to shampoo directly afterward, do so. It won't harm your hair in any way. And don't hesitate to shampoo color-treated hair often. The belief that you shouldn't do so is just a myth. A mild, pH-balanced shampoo is formulated *not* to strip color; what it *will* do is wash out the excessive heaviness of the color to give you a more natural look.

Preparing Hair for Shampooing. Hair should always be thoroughly brushed and detangled before shampooing. Besides making it easier to wash properly, the brushing stimulates the scalp and loosens dry flakes. It's also an easy way to determine whether you have dandruff or other scalp problems. If you use hair spray, brushing will remove most of the stiffness.

· · · · · · · · T·O·O·L·S · · · · · · · · ·
There are two types of brushes to use before shampooing. Whether your hair is straight, curly, kinky, short, medium, or long, a *natural* bristle brush should be used for fine to medium textured hair and/or a sensitive scalp. For medium, coarse, or thick textured hair, a *nylon* bristle brush is best.

· · · · · T·E·C·H·N·I·Q·U·E · · · · ·
Always start at the nape of the neck, working toward the front in sections. Your front hairline and crown hair are most susceptible to breakage, so use the least amount of pressure in these spots. For further stimulation, brush against the growth of your hair while bending at the waist. This not only stimulates your scalp, but increases circulation and gives you a few more minutes of exercise. Always check your brush to see how much hair is lost during brushing. Small amounts are normal, but an excess can be a sign of illness, stress, or improper brushing (see Chapter 17).

HOW TO SHAMPOO

The best part of visiting your hairdresser is having your hair shampooed. It can be a relaxing, luxurious, and stimulating experience. Follow these steps and you'll be able to enjoy the same feeling right at home.

1. Wet your hair well. Don't forget the hairline and nape of the neck. Water should be as warm as possible. This makes the hair cuticles open and stand up—just as warm water opens the pores of your skin for thorough cleansing.
2. Use a minimum amount of shampoo for the first soaping; if a second soaping is absolutely necessary, use only half that amount.
3. When applying shampoo, don't pour it directly onto your head. Try squeezing it into the palm of your hand, then apply to your hair. This lets you control the amount you use. Remember, too much shampoo is hard to rinse out, and it can cause soft, flyaway hair.
4. Dilute any shampoo with water (3 parts water to 1 part shampoo). It'll last longer and save you money.
5. Work the shampoo in, starting on top of the head and working down the length of the hair. Be firm, but not rough. Long hair, bleached hair, or chemically treated hair are especially susceptible to tangles. Erratic, every-which-way motions when you shampoo only result in more tangles. Be sure to massage your scalp with the balls of your fingers. Firmly but gently, rotate the scalp back and forth until it feels tingly.
6. Concentrate around the hairline and neckline areas, where dry flakes usually accumulate. Don't be too rough, though, because wet hair is weak hair and tends to break easily.
7. Rinsing is the most important step, so allow enough time to do a good job. Short hair is easily rinsed under the shower by shaking your head while you separate the sections with your fingers. Medium to long hair needs special rinsing, especially in the thick crown area. Lift small sec-

tions and begin rinsing at the bottom, near the neckline, and work your way up to the crown of the head. The final rinse should be done while bending forward and letting the water penetrate the neckline area. Then stand up, tilt your head back, and let the water hit the front hairline. Add a touch of apple cider vinegar to your rinse water to remove the last traces of any shampoo and to restore your natural pH balance.

8. Now your clean hair is ready for a conditioner (see Chapter 9). (If you're not using one, for whatever reason, go on to step number 10.)

9. Rinse off excess conditioner. Never leave any conditioner on your hair, or it will cause it to be greasy.

10. Finally, end with an invigorating, shine-producing cold water rinse. What does this actually do? Each hair strand is covered with tiny cuticles, much like shingles on a roof. Coloring makes them stand up so the dye can penetrate. Warm water also makes them erect and open. A cold water rinse has a shrinking and closing effect, making the cuticles lie down flat against the hair strand. This creates a smooth, reflective surface against which light bounces to produce an attractive sheen.

Detangling Hair. Hair may be a woman's crowning glory, but after shampooing it can be a mass of knotty, snarled, dripping locks. Wet hair is like elastic and will stretch only so far before it snaps like a rubber band. This breakage leaves ends thin and will eventually result in split ends. But detangling with the proper tools and the correct technique will minimize damage, avoid frustration, and save you time and money.

· · · · · · · · · T · O · O · L · S · · · · · · · · ·
A wide-tooth comb or a rubber-based plastic or nylon bristle brush with widely spaced bristles or bristle clusters are invaluable for untangling your hair. The combs come in a variety of materials, the most common of which is rubber. Avoid the metal types, which are sharp and hard on both hair and scalp. Widely spaced teeth allow more hair to pass through and therefore decrease tugging and breakage. A comb with narrowly spaced teeth, such as a rat-tail style, or a brush with tight bristles should be avoided.

· · · · · T · E · C · H · N · I · Q · U · E · · · · · ·
The single most important rule is to be gentle. Start from the back of the head and work toward the front. Handle only a small section at a time. Lift each section and smooth it completely by starting from the ends and working up toward the roots. If your hair is long and/or chemically treated, it's best to start with a brush and follow up with the comb. Permanent-waved hair must be detangled in very small segments, combing first from underneath and then on top. You can easily stretch a curl when the hair is wet, so if you want curls, comb less and comb gently.

If you hit a knot, use a wide-tooth rake comb and never a regular comb or brush to untangle it. Take the comb tip and gently stroke it through the knot. Don't pull. This will detangle the knot without hair breakage.

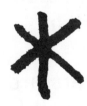
Other Bright Ideas
If you don't have time for a regular wet shampoo or are sick in bed and can't wash your hair, here's a quick and simple solution. Take baking soda or ordinary baby powder and sprinkle it on your brush. Then brush through your hair. It will absorb a certain amount of grime and oil and leave hair cleaner.

Dab cologne or perfume around your hairline to remove excess oil. It'll make you feel refreshed and also smell good.

conditioners

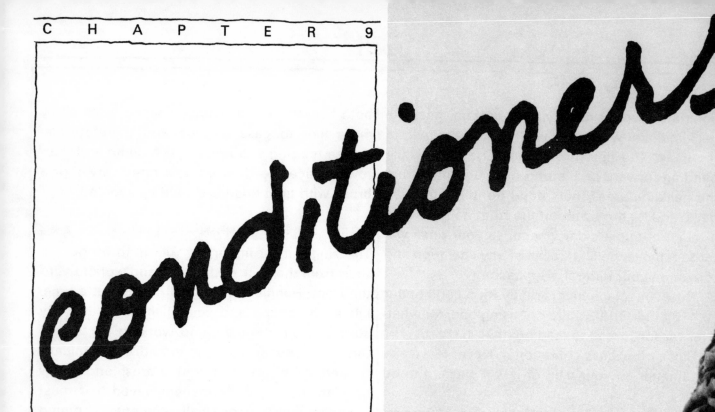

There's an adage that says "Always put back what you take out." That's sound advice not only for the farmer's soil and your savings account, but also for the health of your hair.

Today's instant stylers are also stealers. Between blow-dryers, electric rollers, harsh bleaches and chemicals, hair is robbed of its natural moisture, bounce, and well-being. Heat dries the hair; chemicals change its texture; constant windings over roller spikes break and split it

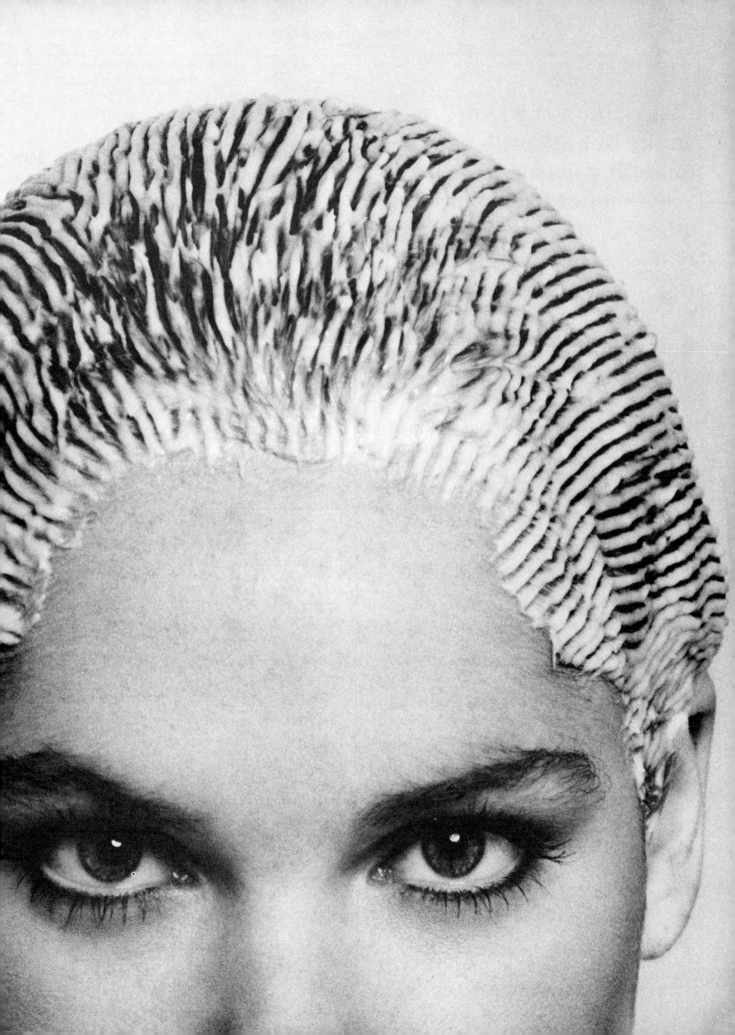

badly. But since I know you're not about to abandon modern conveniences, I ask that you put back a little of what you take out of your hair with *conditioners.* Only regular conditionings restore the hair's health. They put back what nature gave it— and even a little more.

Today's market is flooded with products promising everything from dazzling shine to doubling your hair volume. Don't be misled. Choosing what's right starts with assessing your own specific kind of hair damage and then applying the correct conditioner that will help solve the problem. Here are some tips and pointers to make product selection and proper use of it easier.

First you should know the difference between rinses, conditioners, and deep treatments. They are all different in formulation, and they all work differently and achieve different results.

RINSES

A rinse is simply a product that untangles the hair and has no conditioning effects. In some instances, a rinse can do more harm than help, especially if the product contains paraffin oil or beeswax. What these cream-type rinses do is coat the hair, leaving it with a slick, greasy film. If you insist on a rinse as part of your hair care ritual, find one that is oil-free.

RINSE RECIPES

Here are some of my favorite "home-made" rinses you can put together right in your own kitchen. Each has been tested for its effectiveness, so if you try one, follow the directions and measurements carefully.

SPEARMINT RINSE
for shine and controlling oiliness

Boil 1 quart of water with 3 heaping tablespoons of spearmint leaves. Cool and refrigerate. Use as an after-shampoo rinse—be sure to rinse out excess—for creating great shine and controlling oily hair.

EUCALYPTUS RINSE
for shine and controlling oiliness

Chop 1 large stalk of eucalyptus. Boil in 1 quart of water. Cool and refrigerate. Use as an after-shampoo rinse— rinsing out excess— for beautiful shine and controlling hair oiliness.

THYME RINSE
for dandruff

Boil 4 heaping tablespoons of thyme in 2 cups of water for 10 minutes. Strain and cool. Pour 1 cup over damp, shampooed hair, making sure liquid covers the scalp. Massage in gently. Do not rinse. Makes enough for 2 treatments. Thyme is said to have mild antiseptic properties and can be effective in helping to alleviate dandruff.

CUCUMBER RINSE
for oily hair

Mash 1 whole cucumber in a blender with just enough water to make a paste. Apply to shampooed, towel-dried hair. Leave on for 10 minutes. Rinse well. Excellent for oily hair.

ROSEMARY RINSE
for dull hair

Boil 4 tablespoons of rosemary in 2 cups water for 10 minutes. Strain, cool. Pour 1 cup over damp, shampooed hair. Massage into scalp. Rinse. Rosemary is said to be a stimulant and can help dull, drab, lifeless hair especially during winter months when it's kept under wraps.

SAGE RINSE
for oily hair

Boil 1 tablespoon sage in 1 quart of water. Add juice of 1 lemon. Strain and refrigerate. Use after shampoo rinse, and rinse out excess. A mild astringent rinse that's especially good for oily hair.

LEMON JUICE RINSE
for shine

Squeeze and strain the juice of ½ lemon into 1 cup of cold water and stir. Pour over damp hair. Leave on for 3 minutes. Rinse with cold water. Gives super shine to all hair types.

CAMOMILE RINSE
for blonde hair

Put 10 camomile teabags or 10 tablespoons of camomile tea in 1 quart of water and boil for 10 minutes. Let cool (strain if you use loose tea). Pour over damp, rinsed hair after you shampoo. Do not rinse again. Makes enough for 4 rinses. Adds ash-blonde lights to blonde hair.

CONDITIONERS

Every head needs a conditioner after shampooing, even the oily ones. Hardly anyone escapes the damages we live with: sun, wind, chlorine, chemicals, electricity, even our own perspiration. Recognizing the damage you have is a smart first step in selecting the right conditioner. For example, if you have fine but oily hair, avoid a heavy, creamy conditioner. It only makes fine hair limp, and oily hair oilier. In general, try using a good protein-enriched conditioner. This helps restore healthy hair and protects against most hair abuse while it adds shine and manageability. And since protein coats the hair, slightly increasing hair diameter, it results in more body.

Conditioners come in almost as many formulations as shampoos. Some include lemon, herbs, eggs, minerals. A conditioner is only a temporary restorer of natural oils, but it's a necessary one. Its effectiveness is not determined by the amount of time you leave it on, so don't expect 30-second or 60-second miracles. Conditioners don't penetrate the hair—they only coat the hair strands. For instance, a protein conditioner can help damaged, dry hair by filling in the cracks in the cuticle. In this way it forms a shield around the hair shaft, helping it to retain moisture. Remember, the purpose of a conditioner is not to make hair soft, but to help it stay healthy.

In selecting a conditioner, try to stay away from those brands that require no rinsing out. They often leave hair gummy, and within a few hours you'll wish you had never bothered. I usually suggest three or four different kinds of conditioners and let a client experiment with them. Since each woman's hair reacts differently to products, testing is the only way to find a favorite. As with shampoo, I also recommend you alternate conditioners so that the hair remains responsive to the ingredients. Use one type for two weeks, then switch to another for the next two.

CONDITIONER CHART

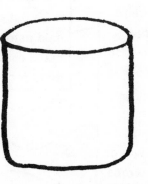

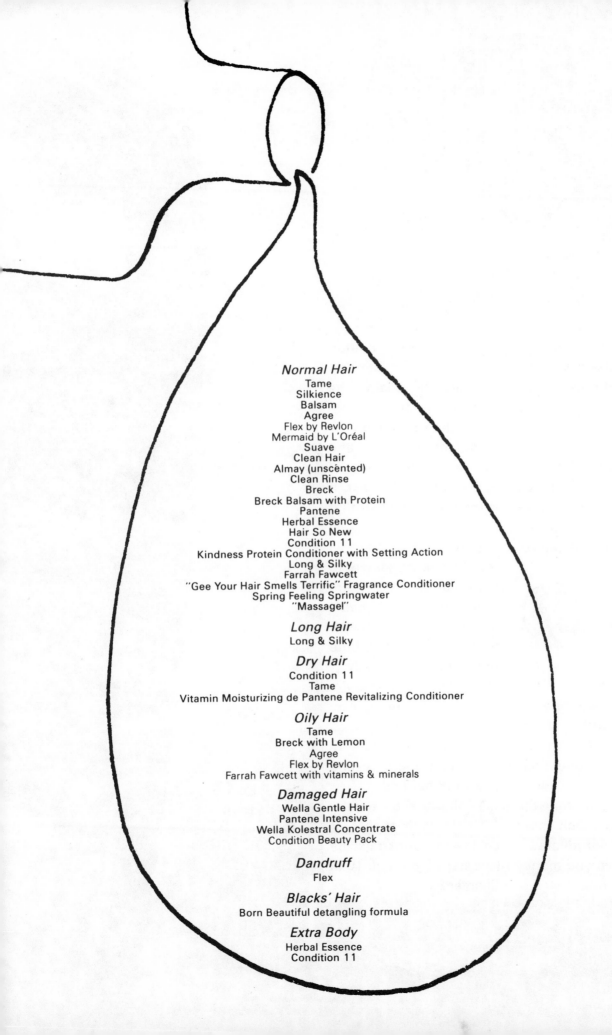

Normal Hair
Tame
Silkience
Balsam
Agree
Flex by Revlon
Mermaid by L'Oréal
Suave
Clean Hair
Almay (unscented)
Clean Rinse
Breck
Breck Balsam with Protein
Pantene
Herbal Essence
Hair So New
Condition 11
Kindness Protein Conditioner with Setting Action
Long & Silky
Farrah Fawcett
"Gee Your Hair Smells Terrific" Fragrance Conditioner
Spring Feeling Springwater
"Massagel"

Long Hair
Long & Silky

Dry Hair
Condition 11
Tame
Vitamin Moisturizing de Pantene Revitalizing Conditioner

Oily Hair
Tame
Breck with Lemon
Agree
Flex by Revlon
Farrah Fawcett with vitamins & minerals

Damaged Hair
Wella Gentle Hair
Pantene Intensive
Wella Kolestral Concentrate
Condition Beauty Pack

Dandruff
Flex

Blacks' Hair
Born Beautiful detangling formula

Extra Body
Herbal Essence
Condition 11

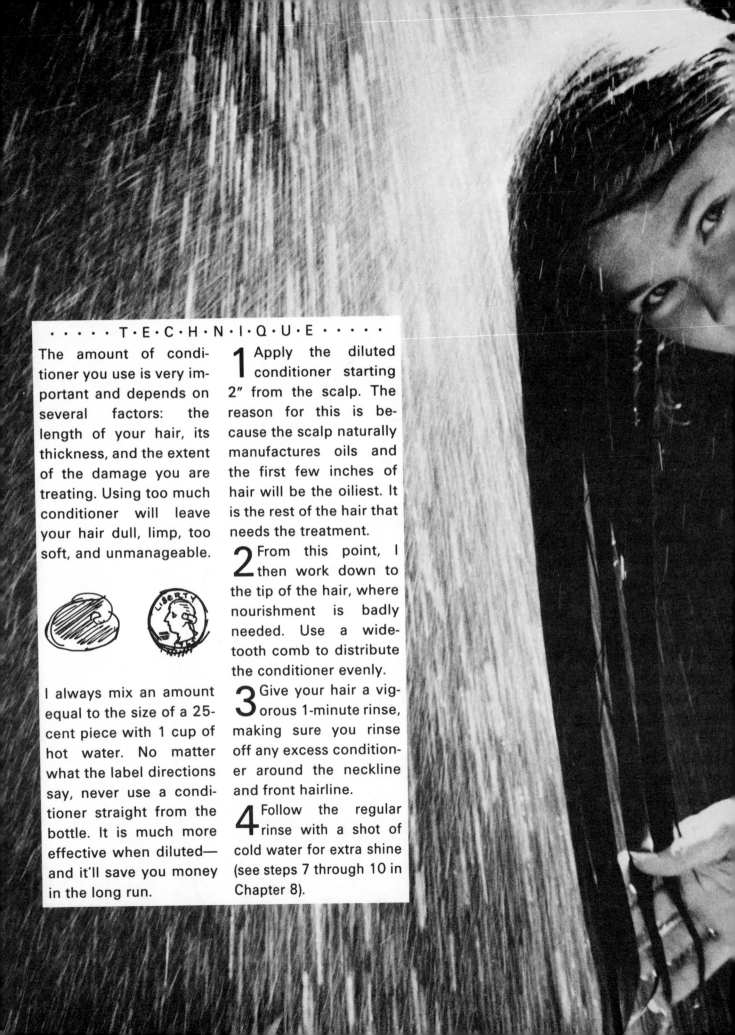

· · · · · T·E·C·H·N·I·Q·U·E · · · · ·

The amount of conditioner you use is very important and depends on several factors: the length of your hair, its thickness, and the extent of the damage you are treating. Using too much conditioner will leave your hair dull, limp, too soft, and unmanageable.

I always mix an amount equal to the size of a 25-cent piece with 1 cup of hot water. No matter what the label directions say, never use a conditioner straight from the bottle. It is much more effective when diluted— and it'll save you money in the long run.

1 Apply the diluted conditioner starting 2″ from the scalp. The reason for this is because the scalp naturally manufactures oils and the first few inches of hair will be the oiliest. It is the rest of the hair that needs the treatment.

2 From this point, I then work down to the tip of the hair, where nourishment is badly needed. Use a wide-tooth comb to distribute the conditioner evenly.

3 Give your hair a vigorous 1-minute rinse, making sure you rinse off any excess conditioner around the neckline and front hairline.

4 Follow the regular rinse with a shot of cold water for extra shine (see steps 7 through 10 in Chapter 8).

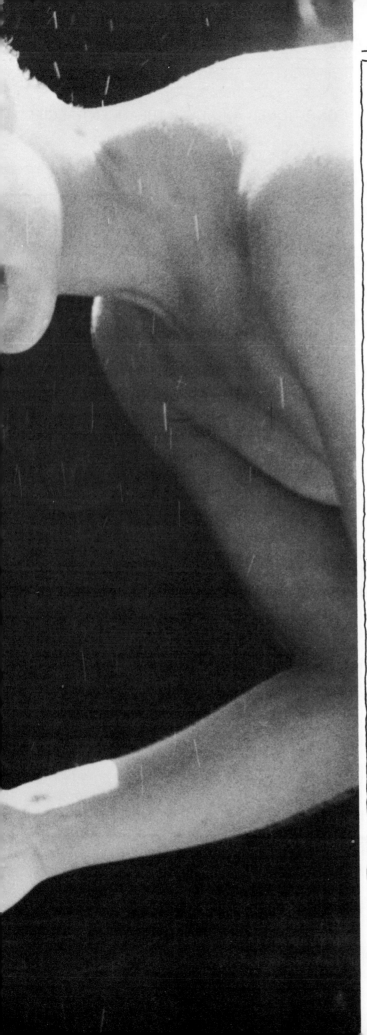

DEEP TREATMENTS

These preparations are specially formulated to penetrate a weak or damaged hair shaft with nutrients that will bring it back to its natural, healthy state. Deep conditioners will not wash out in the next shampoo. Their effect will last up to a month or more.

Clients constantly ask me how often they should have a deep treatment, and the answer to that varies. If the hair is badly damaged because of the chemicals from permanents, straightening, or coloring, I recommend a deep treatment every two weeks. Otherwise, once a month is sufficient. However, during the summer months, if there is an excessive exposure to sun, wind, and water, I suggest a bimonthly treatment.

There are many packaged products on the market that are effective and easy to use. I especially favor some of those sold through beauty supply stores. They give extremely satisfactory results, and you can apply them yourself at home. Use them as directed—or, for an extra boost, try wrapping your head with foil after applying the treatment and sitting under a hair dryer or in the sun for 15 minutes.

For a really beneficial *natural* restorative, I am a particular fan of the pure olive oil treatment, and I've perfected a process, which I call my *Double O Booster*, that I think is the most beneficial—and certainly the least expensive—deep treatment of all.

Double O Booster Technique. Follow these simple directions, and in less than 30 minutes you'll see and feel the difference:

1 Warm pure olive oil on the stove. Use approximately 2 ounces for long hair, 1 ounce for medium-length, and ½ ounce for short hair.

2 With a piece of cotton, apply the oil lightly to the ends of the hair and to those spots that

83

are damaged.

3 Distribute the oil evenly by combing it through the hair with a wide-tooth comb. Try not to touch the scalp if possible.

4 Wrap your head with sheets of aluminum foil.

5 Sit this way in the sun or under a hairdryer or heating cap for 15 minutes. Just as cold water causes the hair cuticles to lie flat, heat causes them to open, allowing the oil to penetrate the hair shaft more effectively.

6 Unwrap and shampoo. Do not try to rinse off the oil first. Apply the shampoo directly to the oil-soaked hair.

7 Rinse and repeat shampoo. This is one of the rare times when I recommend a second soaping. If your hair still remains oily, mix 4 ounces of apple cider vinegar with an equal part of water and rinse with this solution.

The first time you give yourself an olive oil treatment, you'll feel the difference instantly. The penetration of the oil actually restores the hair. And it's completely safe for all types of hair, including that damaged by chemicals or sun. Don't worry about new color being affected by the treatment. Olive oil will not strip color away.

Before you give yourself a Double O Booster, or any kind of deep treatment, be sure to check the condition of your scalp. Scalp condition is not routinely checked at beauty shops, and most people forget this important part of their hair care ritual. For example, oily scalp and dry scalp are common problems that require special treatment and handling. The same holds true for dandruff, which usually occurs on an oily scalp. Of course, dandruff that is accompanied by redness or broken skin might indicate more severe problems, which should be treated by a dermatologist. If you think you might have any kind of scalp problem, don't hesitate to inform your hairdresser about it before he or she does anything to your hair, especially if the process involves chemicals.

CONDITIONER AND DEEP TREATMENT RECIPES

The Double O is not the only treatment I've devised that can be created from products you have in your own home. Any of the following "home recipes" are fun, easy, and effective: just follow the directions closely.

MAYONNAISE CONDITIONER for dry hair

Mix 2 tablespoons of mayonnaise with 2 tablespoons of plain yogurt. Apply to towel-dried hair. Leave on for 10 to 20 minutes. Rinse well.

MAYONNAISE AND EGG CONDITIONER for dry and coarse hair

Mix 4 tablespoons of mayonnaise with 1 whole egg. Apply to dry hair. Comb through, then cover head with aluminum foil. Leave on for 20 to 30 minutes. Shampoo well (two soapings might be necessary). The egg in the mayonnaise acts as an excellent conditioner and moisturizer and will give very dull hair extra shine.

INSTANT EGG CONDITIONER for dry, tired hair

Break 1 egg into a cup, separating the yolk from the white. Add a very small amount of water to the yolk. Apply mixture to hair and leave on for 2 minutes. Rinse off. Follow with cold water splash for super shine.

FLOUR PASTE
for frizzy hair

Make a thin, gooey paste (the consistency of cake batter) from 1 cup of flour and 2 to 3 cups of cold water. Mix until lumps are gone. Apply mixture to dry, unwashed hair, smoothing the mixture and your hair straight back. Leave on for 20 minutes. Rinse thoroughly for about 5 minutes to get all the flour out. Now shampoo hair with one soaping of mild shampoo. Rinse with cool water. Flouring is an ancient recipe that doesn't straighten the hair but smoothes down the scales of the hair shaft, making the hair shinier and more manageable.

VITAMIN E TREATMENT
for damaged hair

Mix contents of 1 400-unit capsule of vitamin E with 1 ounce of soybean oil. With a piece of cotton, apply lightly to the ends and where hair is most damaged. Comb through with large comb to distribute oils evenly. Sit under dryer or heat cap for 15 minutes. Shampoo thoroughly, making sure you apply the shampoo first and not the water—oil and water don't work well together. Rinse. Apply a second soaping. Finish with a cold-water rinse. Vitamin E, proven to have healing properties, adds shine and body to the hair while it dramatically revitalizes a scaling scalp and damaged hair.

WATERCRESS TREATMENT
for oily hair.

Blend a handful of watercress with 1 cup of water in a blender or food processor. Boil the mixture for 10 minutes. Strain out the watercress and cool. Apply carefully to damp, shampooed hair and leave on for 20 minutes. Rinse with cold water. Watercress is a plant rich in iron and phosphorus as well as vitamins A, C, and E. It is said to leave hair bouncy and oil-free.

BEEF-MARROW TREATMENT
for dry, damaged hair

Buy 3 large marrow bones and have butcher crack them in half. Scoop out marrow. Mix with 1 cup of water and bring to boil in a small saucepan. Simmer for 10 minutes. Pour the liquid into cup, straining it through cheesecloth. cool for 2 hours. The marrow will separate from the water and the residue will solidify. Work this mixture in your hands to warm it slightly before putting it on. Apply marrow to dry, unwashed hair with your fingers, one strand at a time, starting at your scalp and working out to the ends. Leave on for 30 minutes. Shampoo with mild shampoo. Rinse with cold water. If your hair is in very bad shape, this treatment is even more effective if you wrap your head with a hot towel. After 15 minutes, rewet the towel in hot water, wring, and wrap your head for another 15 minutes. Then shampoo and rinse. This treatment is used a great deal in Europe and is sometimes fortified with vitamins and applied before a permanent, after coloring, and as a conditioner for dry, damaged, lifeless hair. Beef marrow is rich in natural oils and proteins and gives a beautiful sheen to problem hair.

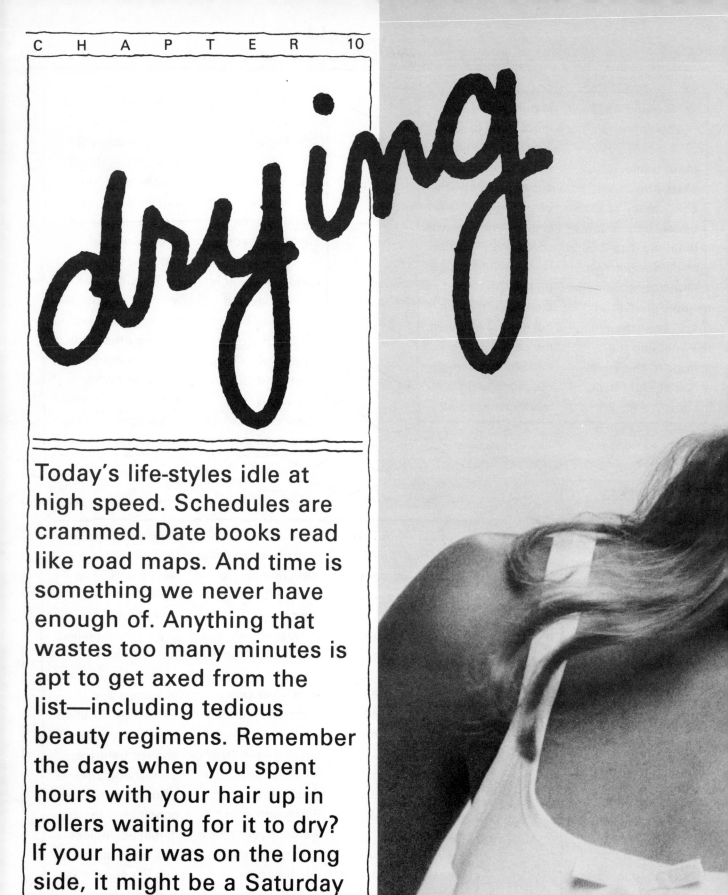

drying

Today's life-styles idle at high speed. Schedules are crammed. Date books read like road maps. And time is something we never have enough of. Anything that wastes too many minutes is apt to get axed from the list—including tedious beauty regimens. Remember the days when you spent hours with your hair up in rollers waiting for it to dry? If your hair was on the long side, it might be a Saturday afternoon affair! Happily, we've packed away that drying agony, along with

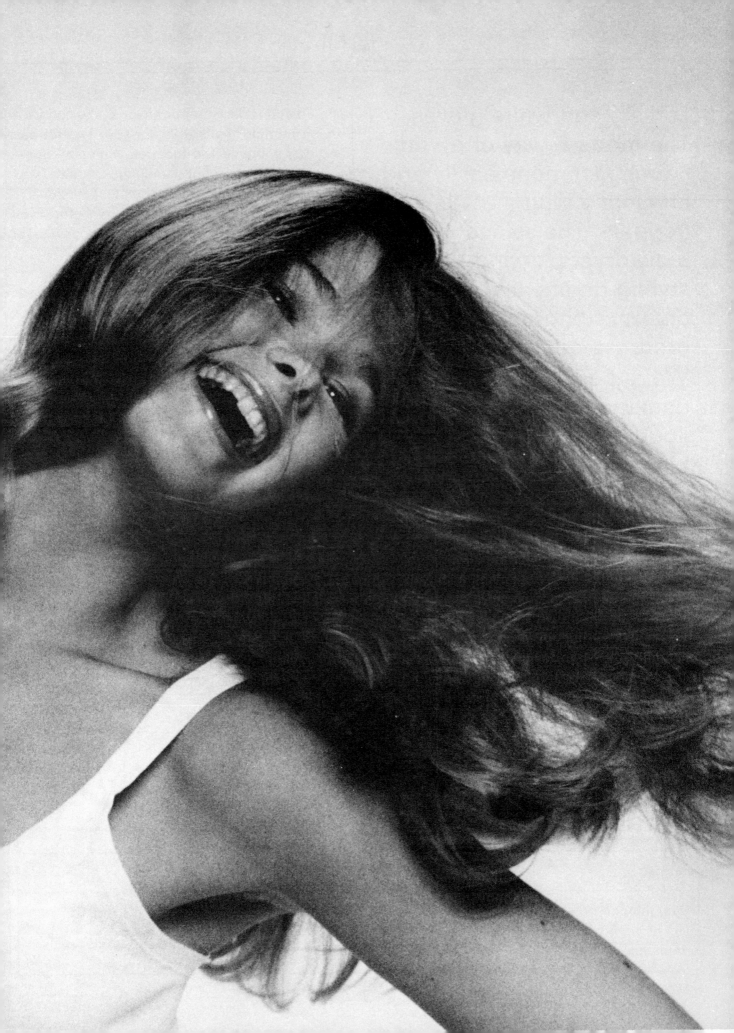

corsets and white gloves. The modern way of drying hair is *fast,* done easily and efficiently with electric gadgets. The selection of blow-dryers, drying combs, styling dryers, and bonnet dryers is enormous. But with progress often comes abuse: We're beginning to see the damage caused by overuse, and improper use, of these high-powered wonders.

The first consideration for anyone is to choose a drying method that's right for your type of hair and that will give you the look you want. Some techniques are fast but damaging. Others are super-easy, but not effective when it comes to styling. Consider the pros and cons before you select. And then learn how to use your new dryer properly.

BLOW-DRYERS

I'd like to discuss blow-dryers first. What's important here is knowing the right wattage to use on your texture hair. The stronger the wattage, the greater the heat that the dryer will produce, and the faster your hair will dry; but an extra few minutes using a lower heat setting will result in healthier hair. Too many watts will create too strong an air flow and will definitely lead to dam-

HAIR TYPE AND TEXTURE	WATTAGE		
	500-600	1000	1200
Fine	✔	✔	
Medium	✔	✔	
Thick		✔	
Coarse			✔
Natural (untreated)		✔	✔
Tinted and Bleached		✔	
Permed		✔	
Straightened		✔	
Hennaed		✔	✔

aged, overblown hair. For **fine hair** I recommend using between 500 and 600 watts only, for **normal to thick hair** 800 to 1000 watts maximum. There are many different opinions on the subject, and often 1200 to 1500 watts are suggested for long hair. But I have too frequently seen hair burned by constant high heat at these settings. If you combine blast-furnace treatment with the continual pulling of a hairbrush that inevitably accompanies drying, your hair can be a disaster in no time.

How to Buy the Right Blow-dryer. When purchasing a blow-dryer, try selecting one with an adjustable power dial, preferably one that offers up to six wattage settings. Usually, the 1000-watts setting is used for straight drying; 750 watts for styling; and 500 watts for touch-ups. You get much more control with these wattage options than with the single-speed model.

Also look for a model that has an automatic thermostat. This will shut off the unit if it overheats and start it again when it's sufficiently cool. Not only is it a good safety factor for the health of your hair, but it also adds to the life of the dryer motor and is less wasteful of electricity.

Other features to look for before buying a dryer: the weight of the model, the length of the cord, the ease of holding it in your hand. And finally, if you travel a lot, the adaptability to European current from 110 to 220. Many travel models are compact, fold-down styles, and cordless versions are even cropping up because wall outlets aren't always handy.

A valuable blow-dryer attachment worth investing in is a diffuser head. Designed like a flattened bowl or a big shower head, a diffuser slips over the barrel end of your dryer. What it does is baffle, or break up, the flow of air so that instead of a blast of heat concentrated on one area, you get diffused warmth that wafts out gently to cov-

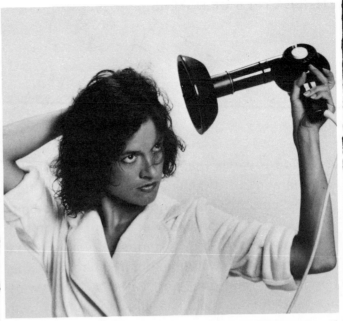

er a larger section of your hair. It seems to get results similar to those of infrared lamps, but without the wait.

How to Use Your Blow-dryer.

1 Remove as much excess water from your hair as possible before you start blow-drying. This saves you time and saves your hair from too much heat.

2 Hold the dryer at least 6" from the scalp; otherwise damage to hair (along with discomfort to ears, neck, and scalp) is guaranteed.

3 Start to dry your hair at the nape of the neck, working your way up the back. Then dry the sides and top of the head.

4 Keep the dryer moving constantly. Concentrating too long on one spot only increases the chance of damage.

5 Alternate between hot and cool settings during the entire process. This reduces hot spots and assures maximum comfort to head and scalp.

Remember, if you blow-dry often, you should use a conditioner after each shampoo. A deep conditioner twice a month is a good idea, especially if your hair is chemically treated; once a month is sufficient for untreated hair.

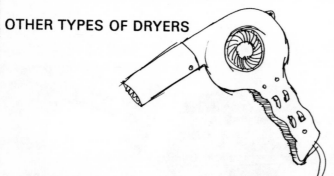

OTHER TYPES OF DRYERS

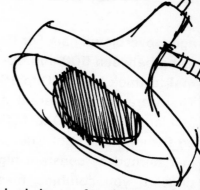

A styling dryer is really a blow-dryer with a full complement of attachments, including air-flow nozzles, combs, and styling brushes. These units are usually larger and heavier to handle than regular blow-dryers. They are most effective at the 1000-to-1200-watt range, but if you're not experienced at using one, start with the lower wattage and follow the instructions provided with the product.

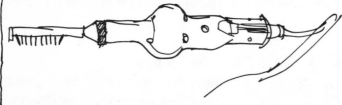

A styling comb is yet another variation and shouldn't be confused with a styling dryer because it has a completely different function. It works more like a curling iron with teeth than like a blow-dryer. Its purpose is to style the hair lightly without any of the lumps, ridges, and bumps that you can get using a brush and hand-held dryer.

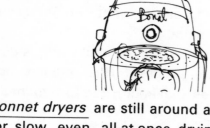

Bonnet dryers are still around and still effective for slow, even, all-at-once drying. They are approximately 250 watts and create an air flow that works over the entire head. Your hair can be set in rollers or simply covered with a net. What's nice about bonnet drying is that your hands are free to do other things.

Infrared lamps are ideal dryers for those with a no-fuss, wash-and-wear cut. It's one of the most natural drying methods because it simulates the sun and works slowly and gently. It is also one of the least damaging of all drying systems available. And the extra bonus is that you don't have to go to the hairdresser for it. Infrared bulbs can be bought at any electrical supply store and screw right into an ordinary light socket. Or, purchase an inexpensive clip-on lamp and use your infrared bulb in it. This will give you total freedom to move around inside or outside the house . . . to sit and dry anywhere you like. Infrared lamp drying is great for loosening permanent-waved, naturally curly, or wavy hair: Use the lamp until your hair is three-quarters dry, then blow-dry. The result will be smooth—but not straight—with lots of soft, feminine movement.

Fresh air is the healthiest drying method. I know that can seem like an impossible choice, given today's tight time schedules, but every now and then you should treat yourself to this luxury. First, though, you may need a new haircut—one of the breezy wash-and-wear styles, for instance. With this you simply shampoo and towel-dry. To help the process along, shake your head and use your fingertips to get rid of the excess water. If you want more fullness and volume, try my **jack-knife drying method:** Bend at the waist and straighten up quickly. Repeat this several times, letting the wind created by the motion dry your hair. Not only will your hair be a few inches fuller, but you might find your waistline getting a few inches trimmer! And you'll certainly find it gets your circulation going.

SPECIAL USES OF HAIRDRYERS

COMPACT

1 for the road (Clairol)—1200-650-300 watts, compact size, folding handle, dual voltage for travel

Pro Max 1200 (Clairol)—1200 watts, heat and air control

Pistol Power 1200 (Conair)—1200 watts, two speeds, two heat settings

Travelair 1200 (Braun)—1200 watts, dual voltage for travel, with plug adapter, air concentrator, travel bag

Gotcha Dry 1000 (Norelco)—1000 watts, styler/dryer with brush and comb attachment

Gotcha Gun 1000 (Norelco)—two heat settings, air concentrator, attachments

Gotcha Gun 1200 (Norelco)—1200 watts, three temperature settings, folds up for travel

DUAL VOLTAGE FOR TRAVEL

Hot Stuff (Clairol)—1200-660-300 watts, dual voltage for travel, adjustable gun dryer, round brush styler, elbow air concentrator, wide-angle concentrator with two snap-in comb attachments

Vagabond (Conair)—1000 watts, dual voltage for travel, two temperature settings, two speeds

Travelair 1200 (Braun)—1200 watts, dual voltage for travel, with plug adapter, air concentrator, travel bag

CURLY OR PERMED HAIR

Supermax Curlytop (Gillette)—1200 watts, gentle air flow designed for curly and permed hair

Curl Dry (Helene Curtis)—attachment

Air Fingers (Conair)—attachment for Conair dryers designed for curly or permed hair

STYLING ATTACHMENTS (INCLUDING AIR CONCENTRATOR)

Son of a Gun (Clairol)—1250 watts, six settings, separate controls for heat and air velocity, air-concentrator attachment

Hot Stuff (Clairol)—1200-660-300 watts, dual voltage for travel, adjustable gun dryer, round brush styler, elbow air concentrator, wide-angle concentrator with two snap-in comb attachments

Pro Style (Conair)— 1200 watts, two speeds, four temperature settings, air-concentrator attachment

Pro Baby 1200 (Conair)—1200 watts, adjustable speed and heat settings, sits on table to free hands

Travelair 1200 (Braun)—1200 watts, dual voltage for travel, with plug adaptor, air concentrator, travel bag

Supermax 2 (Gillette)—200 to 900 watts, adjustable, styler/dryer, power dial, adjustable heat and air flow, four attachments for styling

Supermax 2 Styler/Dryer (Gillette)—1000 watts, detangling and styling comb, finished styling brush

Drying Stick (Schick)—900 watts brush, curlmaker, comb adaptor, round brush attachments, adjustable speed and heat

Gotcha Gun 1000 (Norelco)—two heat settings, air concentrator, attachments

Burst of Air! (Sunbeam)—1200 watts, three speeds, nozzle air concentrator, attachments

1000 Vari-a-matic (Sunbeam)—300 to 1000 watts, adjusts by dial; attachments include two size combs, brush, concentrator nozzle; separate handle for attachments makes two-handed styling possible

SALON-STYLE DRYERS

Dominion (Scovill)—portable console hair dryer, adjustable heat settings

Lady Schick Custom Salon Hair Dryer (Schick)—1400 watts, salon hard plastic hood, adjustable heat settings including those for real and synthetic wigs

BONNET DRYERS

Bonnet Hair Dryer (General Electric)—four temperature settings

Bonnet Dryer (Sunbeam)—bonnet, four temperature settings

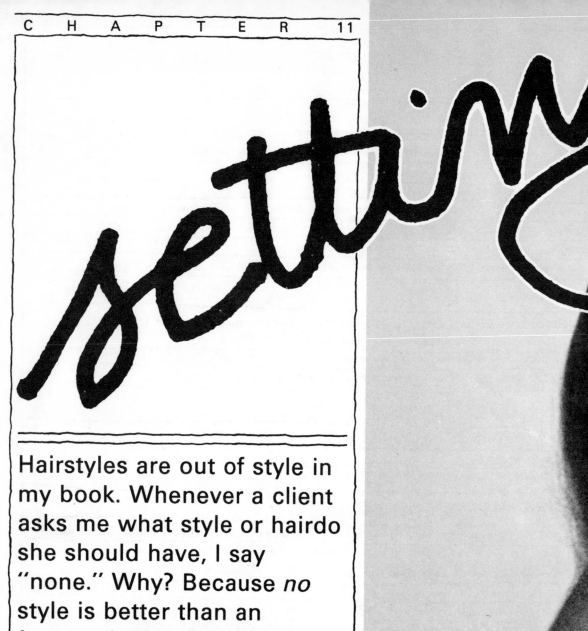

setting

Hairstyles are out of style in my book. Whenever a client asks me what style or hairdo she should have, I say "none." Why? Because *no* style is better than an *imposed* style—especially one that doesn't suit you. I'd rather see you develop a hair *look,* a line, a shape that's right and natural for you. A look that's as individual as you are. Working with each feature—the face shape, the overall body image—that's what counts, and that's what creates a great look. With this system you never make

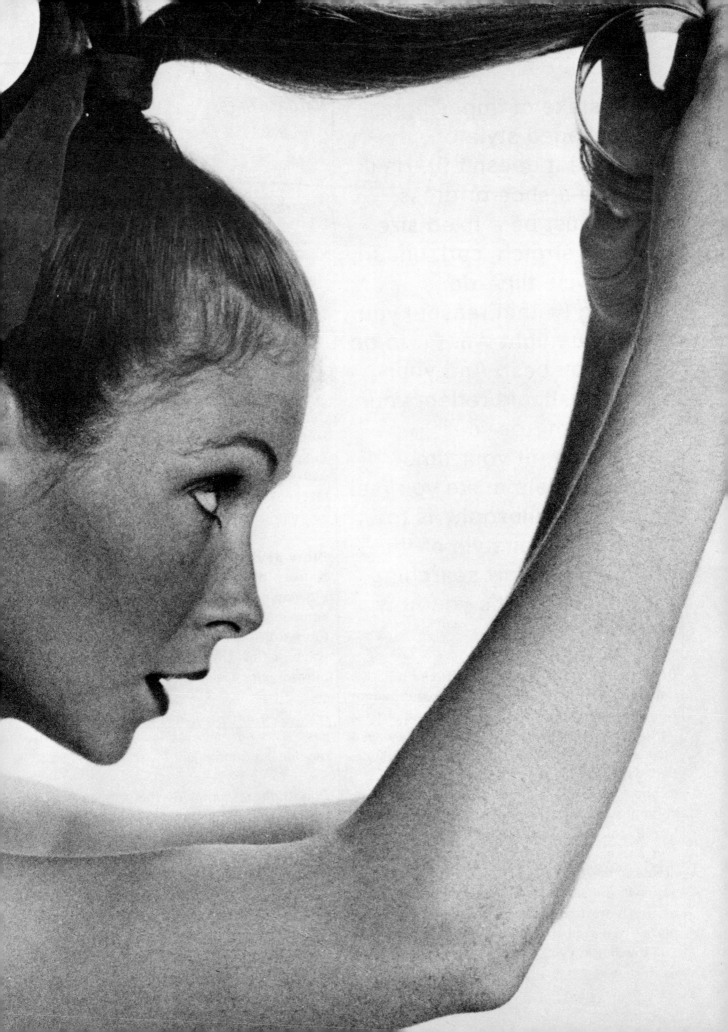

the mistake of imposing a prepackaged style on someone it doesn't fit. Hair isn't like a shoe or dress, which must be a fixed size. Hair can stretch, curl, uncurl, wave, twist, flip—do anything (within reason) you think you might want it to do to suit you best. And your hair look should reflect your life-style, mirror your personality, fit your time schedule, help make you feel good. My philosophy is to forget the "hairstyle of the month" and start searching for the look that's you now. Here's how.

Begin by understanding your hair. Learn its limitations. Know its texture, Evaluate your haircut. Consider whether your hair is processed or treated (permed, straightened, colored, body-waved, etc.). All of these factors affect susceptibility to curl, degree of blow-dry heat necessary, etc. In short, they can dictate the most appropriate setting system to help you achieve your preferred look. Here are some of the most common and popular setting systems, ways to help you create some of the best hair looks ever—all by yourself. But remember, none of them are forever. Try more than one method. Experiment. Explore. That's all part of the learning process— and it will bring you terrific results.

NATURAL SETS:	Blow-drying
	"Helicopter" se
	"Wraparound" se
	Hair rolling
	Rollers and pincurls
CHEMICAL SETS:	Permanent wave
	Body wave
	Curly wave
	Straightening

NATURAL SETS

I call a "natural set" any method of setting your hair that doesn't involve chemicals. It can be done with rollers and pincurls or the more free form methods, including wrapping or twisting. Cut and hair length will have a considerable effect on how well all these methods work for you. But no matter what method you use, always start with your hair combed or brushed straight back (except for bangs). This will give a fuller effect to every finished look.

Blow-drying. This is probably the most popular way of creating hair looks today. Using a blow-dryer to get your look need not be a long, complicated process. Too many women work too hard at putting in or taking away a curl, a wave, a flip. I have several tips to help make blow-drying easier and more successful.

Roll more and pull less during the entire process. This not only produces better results, but reduces hair damage.

Don't fight it, join it. By that I mean you should try to follow the natural growth and flow of your hair, and not force it to go where it doesn't want to go. Also, part your hair where it falls naturally. Here's the best way to find that natural line: Brush the top of your hair straight back. Place your hand on the crown of your head and push it forward toward the front hairline. Wherever your hair splits is its natural part. If you have a

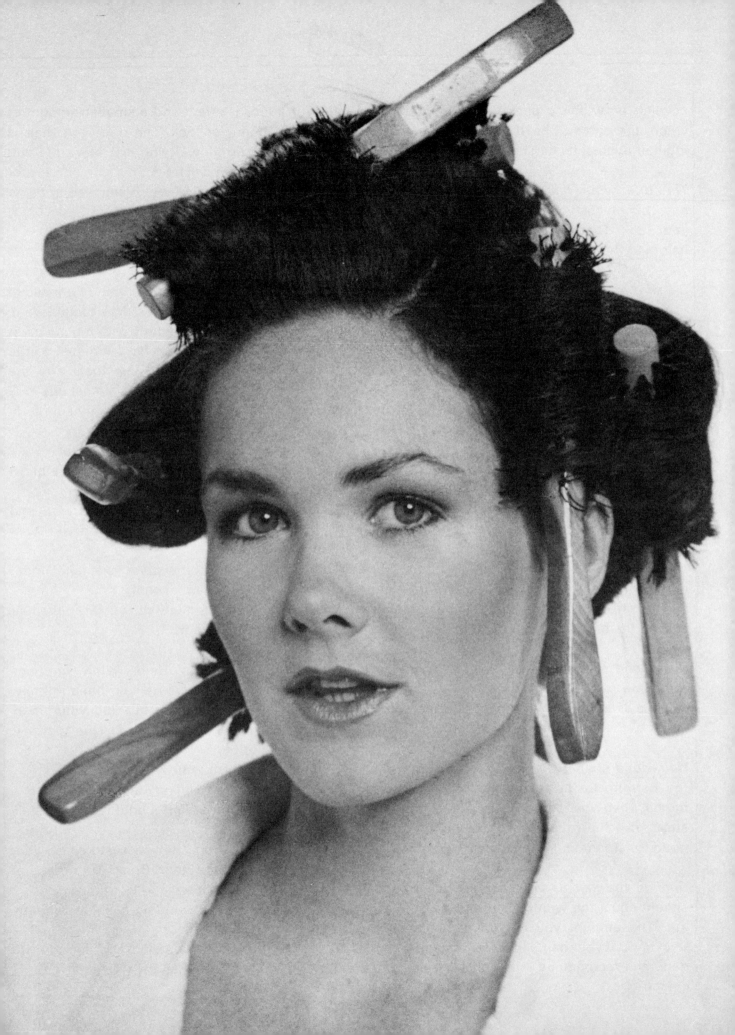

cowlick or widow's peak, let them determine where the part will be. If you don't, you're forcing hair against its natural growth.

The drier your hair is to start with the better. This means you'll need less heat to achieve your look. Therefore, the less damage to your hair over the long haul.

Be sure you are using the right size and type brush. (See Brush Chart in Chapter 7.) There's one basic guideline to follow in brush selection: The smaller the brush you use, the curlier the look; the larger the brush, the smoother, looser, and straighter the look.

Shape is more important than bristle in blow-dry brushes.

Full round shapes are available in a large size to give more fullness, especially at the bottom. The medium size gives more body on top and a tighter curve on the bottom. It's a good size for layered cuts and for making short, curly hair smoother. The small round type is perfect for a curly look. It's also what you'll want for creating special effects and for curling those short hairs around the hairline.

Oval round shapes will give the classic pageboy look. One of the newer designs in this type of brush is a flattened round shape that lets you get closer to the scalp for a less full look.

Half round shapes are good for a fuller effect at the bottom; to flip up hair; to get wide-swept bangs when you want just the tips to flip up instead of a full round look. The medium size is good for smoothing out curly and short hair.

Section the hair as you shape it. Each section should equal the width of the brush you are using. The amount you roll up depends on the thickness of your hair and the effect you want. In general, I recommend rolling a larger section of hair for a looser effect and a smaller amount of hair for a bouncier look. The drier your hair is when you begin blow-drying, the more the curl or wave you put in will hold. This is important for loose body-wave styling, but it can also apply to naturally wavy or curly hair.

How to Get Great Blow-dry Looks. By and large, blow-drying makes curly or wavy hair look straighter, and if the look you want is a mass of curls, this may not be the best way to achieve it. You can, however, create curls with a blow-dryer and a small round brush; in fact, with just a little practice and patience, the best tools and the right technique, you can achieve almost *any* look you like with a blow-dryer. Here is my simple *5-step method to effective blow-dry setting:*

1. Towel-dry hair to remove excess water.
2. Bend forward and finger-dry hair with a blow-dryer until hair is almost dry.
3. Take a section of hair, smooth it out, and wrap it around brush in the direction you want the curl to go.
4. Direct heat from blow-dryer over and under the wrapped hair, then let cool.
5. When hair is completely cool, unwrap the hair from brush and shake it.

Blow-dryer emergency. Help! What happens when you're all set to create your beautiful new hair look for the big night out and your trusty blow-dryer goes on the fritz? *Don't worry.* There's a solution.

1. Towel-dry hair to remove excess water.
2. With your brush, gently direct hair into a shape you like, smoothing it until it's completely dry.
3. Bend forward from the waist and brush your dried hair toward the floor. Brush 10 strokes or more. This gives fullness.
4. Swing back into a standing position, smoothing the top hairs.
5. Hair will look freshly styled and nobody will know your blow-dryer standby was *you!*

Classic Blow-dry Looks. There are really three classic looks from which scores of variations spring. Master the following blow-drying methods and you can create a wide variety of hair fashions for yourself.

1. "Pageboy" Look: First, your hair should be all the same length and just touching your shoulders. The hair can be parted anywhere (center, off-center, to either side). Now take your brush (the size of which will depend on the texture and length of your hair) and for more bounce and fullness, hold the side section of hair out from the face and wrap it around the brush (toward the head). Follow the same forward movement all the way around.

2. "Angled-away" Look: Hair should be cut at an angle all around the head. The length will vary depending on your features. Hair should be blow-dried away from the face and always in the same direction (the one you want). Hold the side section of hair up and roll back vertically away from the face. Top section of hair should be rolled straight back for a more versatile look. Be sure to check that you're using the correct size and shape brush.

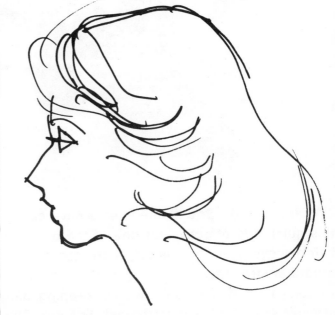

3. "Upswing" Look: Hair should be cut at a slight angle at the bottom (to make the ends turn up more easily) and can be any length, from chin-length to above the shoulder. The part can be anyplace. For more fullness, hold the side section of hair straight out. Using a large brush, place on topside of hair and roll up. Apply heat over and under the rolled section. Continue the same upswing movement all around the head.

97

"Helicopter" Set. A natural straightener, this works best on shoulder-length or longer hair. It's a 30-minute process from start to finish and will leave your hair sleek, straight, and lovely.

1. Start with damp hair. Bend head down and pull hair into a ponytail on crown of head. Tie it in place by making 2 or 3 turns with a scarf or stocking.

2. Comb and smooth out ponytail and then separate into three sections.

3. Using three rollers (the larger the roller the looser the curl), roll center section in the direction of the forehead, the other two angled toward the back of the ears.

4. Wrap a net over everything.

5. Sit under dryer for 15 to 20 minutes (longer if your hair is thicker).

6. Brush out for a fabulous straight look.

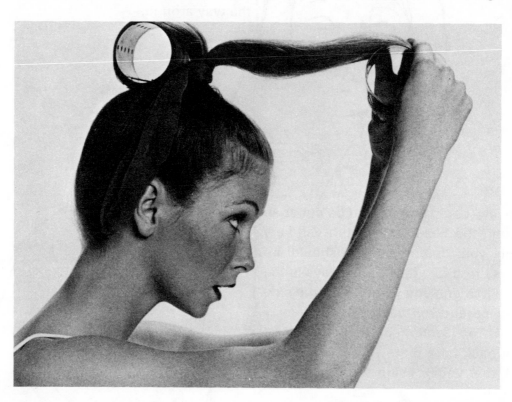

"Wraparound" Set. Some clients have called this quick and effective set one of the greatest hair discoveries of the century. I created it to be a natural straightener for longish to long, wavy to curly hair. And it really works, keeping hair straight even in the most humid weather. The "Wrap" is so easy because you actually use your head as a roller. Here's how.

1. While the hair is wet, section off the crown hair into 3 parts, and roll each one backward on a jumbo roller (juice cans will do the job well). This adds height.

2. Starting from the front of one side, take small vertical sections of hair and comb each across the forehead and as far around the back as it will go. Where it ends, clip in place.

3. Keep doing this with each section—wrapping and smoothing, always in the same direction. Remove clips from underneath as you work; the hair will stay in place without them, and clips will only create ridges.

4. Smooth out any wrinkles.

5. Soak end papers with water and wipe hair to keep any flyaways in place. What you should have at this point is a shiny, sleek cap of hair.

6. Sit under the dryer or out in the fresh air until hair is bone-dry.

7. Brush out. You'll be amazed how straight and swinging and stylish your hair will look.

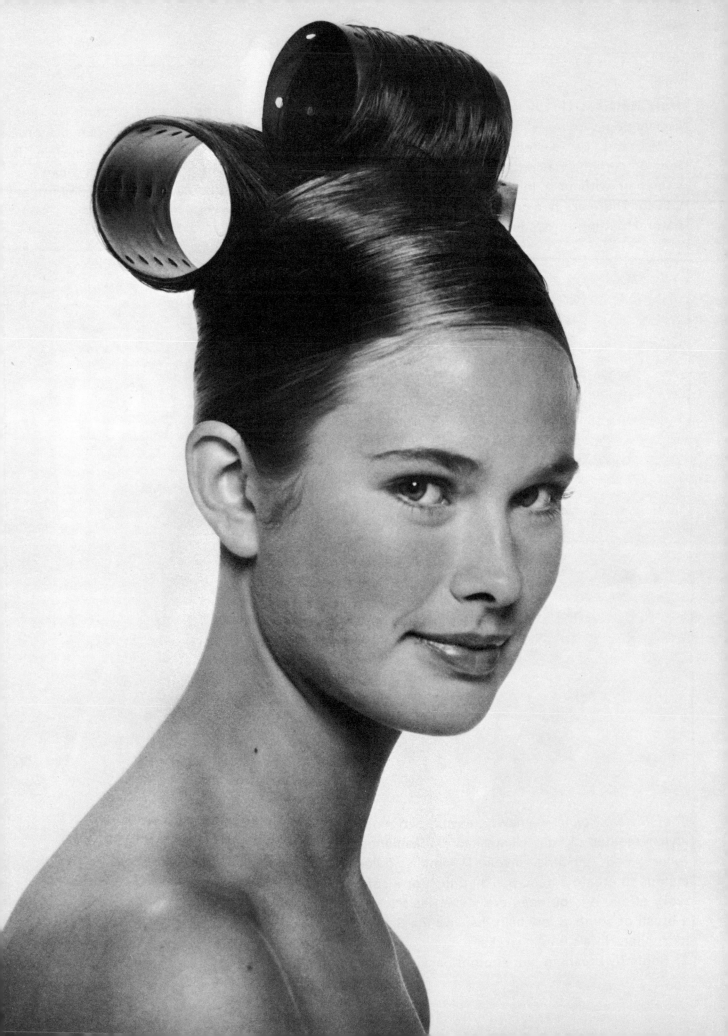

Hair Rolling. This is not to be confused with conventional roller setting. Both the "Riviera Roller" and "Le Twisteur" represent a new system of curling, waving, and giving bounce to your hair without a lot of the fuss it once involved. There are two great advantages to these natural setting procedures: You can perform them on dry hair as an easy solution for quick spot sets; and you can actually wear the ornaments the sets are done with. (The specially designed ornaments from Riviera can be purchased in beauty supply shops, department stores, and some drugstores.)

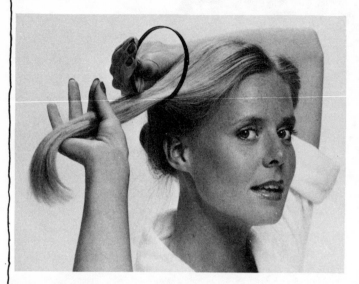 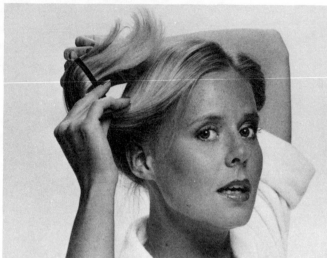

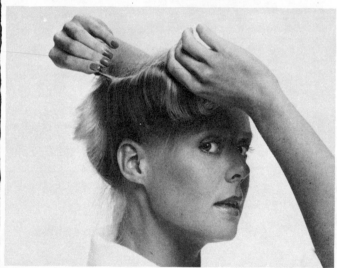 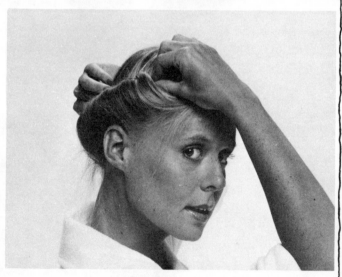

The "Riviera Roller"—a newer, easier, and more stylish method of hair rolling than old-fashioned rollers and pincurls—involves simple roller clamps to create a neat, polished look or a soft, wavy effect. All you need are some basic tools: a brush or comb, a few hairpins, and the Riviera hair roller. Here's how it works.

1. Begin by brushing hair straight back. Section hair into equal parts. Open the "roller" and slip through a section of hair.

2. Close clamp halfway down the hair section. Start rolling.

3. Wind hair in an upward motion to the desired height and position above ear. Secure with hair pins if necessary.

4. Repeat on other side to complete the effect.

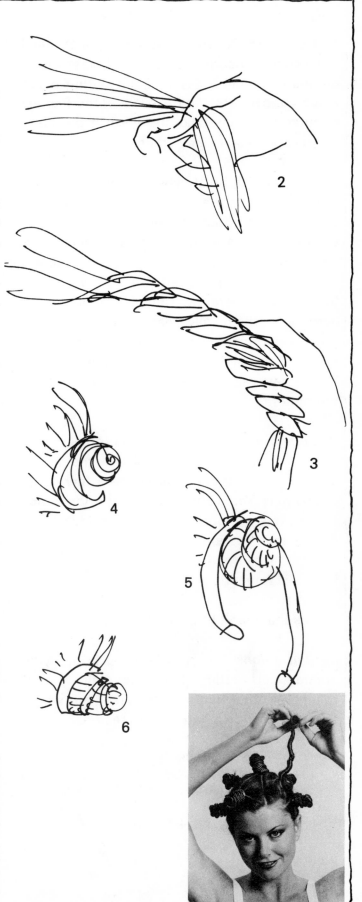

"*Le Twisteur*" is a fabulous new natural method of setting done without any clips, pins, conventional rollers, curling irons, or chemicals. The secret: "Twistesse" ornaments by Riviera. From start to finish the whole process takes 20 minutes, and the set will last from shampoo to shampoo. Though it's ideal for dry hair (it gives a looser look), Le Twisteur can be done on damp hair. This will take 8 to 15 minutes of drying time depending on the thickness of your hair, and it will create a firmer set. Just follow the illustrations on this page.

Le Twisteur is best done on long, layered hair, on medium-length hair, or on long hair. It is excellent on fine hair because it gives body and volume. The larger the section of hair twisted, the larger the wave will be, but the minimum number of sections you should use is six. If you want a very curly look, just twist more sections.

What's such fun about Le Twisteur is the original look it has while it's setting the hair. In fact, it's so great you can literally "wear" the hair ornaments for an evening of disco, skating, or partying. It's also an ideal solution at the beach and for after-beach setting.

These sets, as noted, can be done with wet *or* dry hair, though you'll get a looser effect if your hair is dry when you set it. One precaution: Be careful not to "bake" your already dry hair with a blow-dryer. If you feel you want a more definite set for your hair, try dampening it with a wet comb or brush, or misting it with an atomizer—or even a plant sprayer!

Rollers and Pincurls. As I mentioned earlier, rollers and pincurls may seem old-fashioned in comparison with today's instant-setting modern electrical gadgets, but believe me, the few extra minutes they may take are worth it because of the reliable results they create.

Rollers (*regular,* brush-type, or electric) can leave ridges. A way to prevent this is to zigzag the part as you section hair for rolling. A rat-tail comb works best because it separates the hair strands easily and neatly. Electric rollers, often preferred because they're quick and curl well, will dry your hair if used constantly. They are particularly disastrous on chemically treated hair. So I suggest you use end papers every time you set with hot rollers. This will give your hair some protection. But in general, the less you use electric rollers the better.

Pincurling, on the other hand, is totally safe for the hair. Part of its simplicity is the minimal amount of equipment you need—a few clips or bobby pins. Years ago I took great pride in doing pincurl sets without using any clips. I twirled and curled each section in such a way that it would stay put until dry. But if you don't feel like playing artist, pincurls are great "spot" sets and are especially effective for those short hairline pieces that won't fit over rollers or brushes.

Setting lotions. You may be used to applying a commercial setting lotion to help pincurls, rollers, or other natural sets "take" but why not try one of my own home-made recipes?

SETTING LOTION RECIPES

• *SUGAR WATER*
Dissolve 2 tablespoons of plain sugar in 1 quart of warm water. Use as a setting lotion on damp hair.
• *RICE WATER*
Save the rinse water from cooking rice. Cool and use as a setting lotion.

CHEMICAL SETS

Permanent Wave. Remember those nightmare days when Mother dragged you to the beauty salon for the hair miracle of the month? The long, painstaking process call a "perm" took hours and then left you with the worst case of frizzies ever. Applying and controlling the old-style solutions was as unreliable as the weather. You just never knew what the result was going to be. Timing was split-second. Spilled chemicals burned. Hair breakage was common, and bleached hair wasn't even in the running because the perm's performance was so erratic and unpredictable. But times have changed. Today's permanent waves, now called body waves or curly waves, have been improved both in quality and technique to give thousands of women new freedom. However, the outcome still rests in the hands of the person giving the permanent. Modern perms are mostly wash-and-wear wonders. And thanks to new electronic developments, pH-balanced solutions, and postperm conditioners, waves can be given to practically anyone, including women with bleached hair.

How perms work. The cortex layer of hair is made up of long molecular chains. These fibers are held together by cross-links. In order to alter the hair from straight to curly (or curly to straight), the configuration of these links must be broken or released. During a perm, chemicals are applied to the hair to start the releasing action. Hair is wrapped on rods specially selected to produce the desired wave pattern. When the hair is wound on rods, more chemicals are applied and a specified time period elapses during which the hair's structure becomes more pliable. The ropelike fibers within the hair shaft change and take on the configuration of the rod. This is the processing time, and it will vary from head to head depending on the hair's porosity. This is why timing is so important in the permanent-wave process. Porous hair, for example, can be processed in from 2 to 4 minutes, while more resistant hair can take much longer. In order for the hair to keep its new curly pattern, the broken bonds must be re-formed when the hair has taken its new shape. This is accomplished by the neutralizing process. The neutralizer is applied while hair is still on the rod. The neutralizer forms new bonds and has a shrinking or hardening effect on the cortex layers of the hair. When rebonding is complete, the waves are permanent.

What about home permanents? Getting good results with do-it-yourself permanents at home is difficult. Many factors—having the right cut, the right hair texture, the right rollers in the right pattern, the right perm solution and product—come into play that can make the difference between disaster and success. I would suggest that you go to your salon and watch a trained expert at work. I know this won't guarantee you excellent results, but the odds improve as you become better educated about the process. Remember, most hair damage comes from correcting expensive mistakes.

Body Wave. Basically, this type of permanent adds form and volume to limp, stringy hair so that it moves with you instead of clinging to your scalp. After a body wave, fine hair actually looks and feels thicker; wiry and coarse hair will be more pliable and manageable. Blow-drying lends added fullness to a body wave.

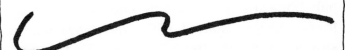

Curly Wave. A curly wave is similar to a body wave. The differences are with regard to the size and amount of rods and rollers on the head and the haircut you have. The more rods or rollers used, the more curl you get. The smaller the rods, the tighter the curl. A curly wave needs a more layered cut than a body wave so as to emphasize the mass of curls.

The beauty of either a body wave or a curly wave is the complete freedom it gives you. After shampooing, for example, just towel-dry, shake your head, and that's it. No fuss or hassle about the set, the weather, the humidity. You wash it and wear it—that's it! On the average, a good perm should last three to six months. Let it grow out if you don't want another perm, but if you decide on this, have your hair shaped so the grow-out stage will look good.

Straightening. If misused, straightening solutions can be the worst chemicals ever to touch your hair. And the chances of damage are great, since most salons use the same strong solution on all hair—regardless of type and texture. The right solution must be applied or damage can be considerable. Try a "strand test" if you're not sure about how the straightening will react on your hair. Have your stylist test the solution on a few strands of your hair, preferably on the top of your head, where the hair is weakest. If these survive, the chemicals in the solution won't harm the rest of your hair.

What a straightener does. A straightener makes hair more manageable. It works exactly the way a permanent wave works, but straightens instead of curling. If you try to make your frizzy

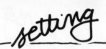

hair bone-straight, you may end up with more frizz than you started with. The more hair is straightened, the drier it becomes. Breakage occurs and instant frizz is almost guaranteed. If your hair is kinky or frizzy and you want a straightening, don't expect your hair to dry smooth on its own. You'll still have to blow-dry it or set it to complete the look.

Mild vs. strong solutions. A mild solution takes out about 70 percent of the curl and leaves in bounce and body. It should be used on chemically treated, fine, and wavy hair. It also adds that extra control you need for humid summer months. During the winter your hair may not be as wavy, and may need less straightening.

A strong solution leaves hair dead straight and without any bounce. It will cause more damage and dullness than mild solutions. Only strong, wiry, or kinky hair should be treated with a strong solution. But if such hair is chemically treated, then the time the chemicals are left on the hair should be reduced. Never use a strong solution on fine or color-treated hair.

With all straightening processes, follow directions explicitly and watch your clock. Timing is very, very important. Be extremely careful around the hairline and top areas where too strong a solution will cause breakage. The hair on the back of your head is stronger and more resistant, so apply straightener to the back first.

PERMANENTS FOR SPECIFIC HAIR TYPES

Color-Treated Hair
Lilt Milk Wave Style Kit (for color-treated hair)
Rave Soft Perm (gentle even for color-treated hair)
Toni Silkwave Gentle (for color-treated or easy-to-wave hair)
L'Oréal Extra Body Perm (protein perm for color-treated hair)

Hard-to-Wave Hair
Lilt Delux Style Kit (super strength for hard-to-wave hair)
Toni Silkwave Super (for hard-to-wave hair)
L'Oréal Extra Body Perm (protein perm for hard-to-wave hair)
Ogilvie Home Permanent (extra body and set)

Regular Hair
Lilt Delux Style Kit (regular strength for normal hair)
Lilt Foam-on Style Kit
Toni Silkwave Regular (for normal hair)
L'Oréal Extra Body Perm (protein perm for normal hair)
Ogilvie Home Permanent (regular body and set)
Rave Extra Curly Soft Perm
Ogilvie Precisely Right Body and Styling Wave
Ogilvie Soft Body Wave with conditioners

HAIR STRAIGHTENERS FOR SPECIFIC HAIR TYPES

Color-treated Hair
Radiance Permanent Creme Relaxer Fine
(for fine, easy-to-straighten, or tinted hair)
Radiance Permanent Creme Relaxer Regular
(for normal, medium-textured, or tinted hair)
Realistic Permanent Creme Relaxer Mild
(for color-treated—not bleached—fine hair)
Realistic Styling Perm
(for color-treated hair)

Regular Hair
U.N.C.U.R.L. Conditioner and Uncurler
(for relaxing locks)
Curl Free
(natural curl relaxer)
Radiance Permanent Creme Relaxer Regular
(for normal, medium-textured, or tinted hair)
Realistic Permanent Creme Relaxer Regular
(for normal, medium-textured hair—not bleached or tinted)
Realistic Styling Perm (for normal hair)
Revlon Curl Relaxer
(for all types of hair except bleached)

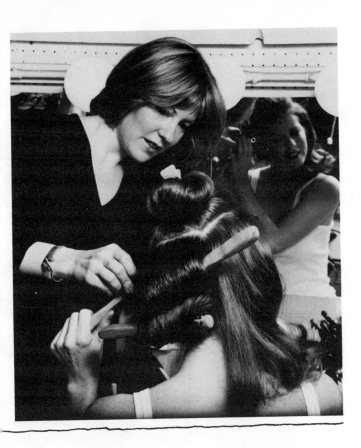

For Uncurly Results
Lilt Bodywave (for uncurly hairdos)
Toni Silkwave (all body-no curl for all hair types; total conditioning)
Toni Lightwaves (gentlest perm that can't overcurl)

Gray or White Hair
Toni Silkwave Silver (curl for gray or white hair)

Between Perm Touch-ups
TipToni Silkwave (touch-up for all hair types)
SupPerm Reinforcing Conditioner for Permed Hair
(the supplement between perms)

Blacks' Hair
Ultra Sheen Permanent Creme Relaxer
(mild strength for delicate hair)
Ultra Sheen Permanent Creme Relaxer
(super strength for stubborn, hard-to-relax hair; with protein)
Ultra Sheen Permanent Creme Relaxer
(regular strength for normal hair)
Curl Out Plus Creme Hair Relaxer Kit

Delicate or Fine Hair
Radiance Permanent Creme Relaxer Fine
(for fine, easy-to-straighten, or tinted hair)
Realistic Permanent Creme Relaxer Mild
(for color-treated—not bleached—fine hair)
Realistic Styling Perm
(for fine or limp hair)

Difficult-to-straighten Hair
Radiance Permanent Creme Relaxer Super
(for coarse, resistant hair)
Realistic Permanent Creme Relaxer
(for resistant or coarse—not bleached or tinted—hair)

coloring

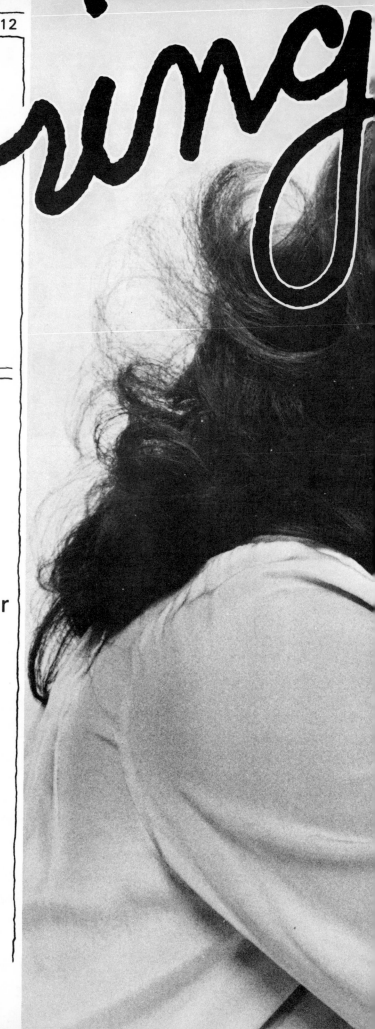

We see our world in color. And we live it that way, too. Color psychologists will tell you their research shows that extroverts traditionally prefer warm, intense colors like reds and yellows, while introverts pick cooler, calmer shades. So if color preferences can paint your personality, let's take a closer look at hair color.

Sometimes, no matter how healthy, clean, or bouncy your hair is, you feel dissatisfied with the way it looks. Something's missing. You need a lift. That's when you first think of coloring

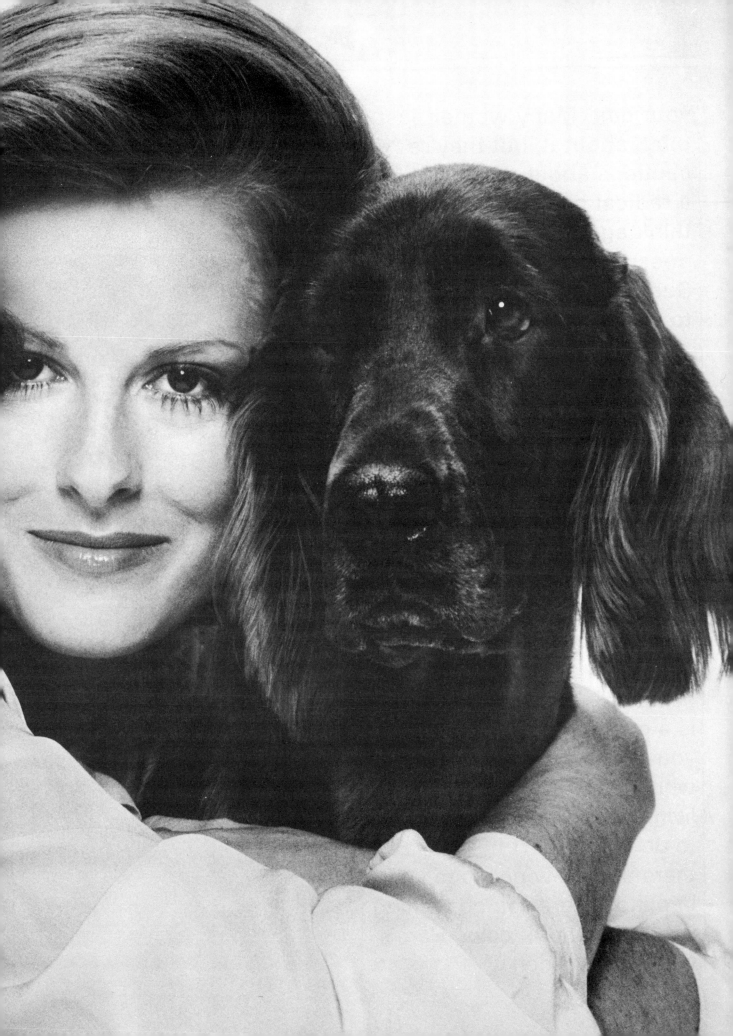

your hair. Many women just think about it, but they're cautious about making such a radical change. If that's you, think again. A color change doesn't have to be radical. Subtle changes can add a lift to your personality as well as to your appearance. Maybe a few red highlights in your drab brown hair are all you need to perk up your skin tone and brighten your eyes. Or covering that gray will boost your confidence while it subtracts a few years from your age. Or adding some golden streaks to a faded blonde head may make you feel as if you spent a glorious summer in the sun. Yes, color is a great way to give all of you—not just your face—a whole new way of looking and living. So my advice to you is to do it and don't hesitate! But there are a few points to keep in mind before you go rushing into the world of color. Here's what to consider:

1 *Your age.* Believe it or not, the normal aging process changes hair texture, causing the hair shaft to thicken. This is important to remember, because it can make hair resistant to certain chemical processes and hair colors.

2 *Attitude toward age.* Weigh your feelings and think about just how you want to look. Many women prefer to look their age, while others don't. If you want to stay looking years younger you might consider hair coloring. But remember two basics: Darker shades add years; lighter shades subtract years.

3 *Climate.* Consider where you live. It can affect hair color. Heat, humidity, and perspiration will oxidize color (cause it to fade) more than the sun itself. So weather and climate are important factors to think about.

4 *Life-style.* Know it and be honest with yourself about it. For example, know how much time your schedule will permit you to spend having your hair colored and how much of your budget you can allocate for the process. Unfortunately, once you've found that perfect shade, it does not last forever. Return trips to the salon and touch-ups are necessary unless you decide you'll allow your original shade to grow back (in which case you have a whole other set of complications). Sometimes these visits can take up an entire afternoon, and for the busy businesswoman, time conflicts are bound to develop. Also, if you're watching your budget you should find out a few facts before you choose a color: a) how long the color will last; b) what it will look like while it's growing out; c) how much the initial visit and the return trips will cost. Don't be embarrassed to discuss price ranges. A good colorist should inform you how to save money. Since prices are usually based on hair length and the amount of work done, estimates are given after a personal consultation.

5 *Skin tone and eye color.* Study them carefully. They are two vital aspects of your face you just can't change. And because they are constant givens, they can be used as color guides in determining what shade of hair will work best for you. I have developed a special skin and eye color guide to help you. Try going through the guide, located at the end of this chapter, to see if you can spot your type.

6 *Degree of change.* Determine just how far you want to go in altering your looks. The words "blonde" and "brunette" encompass a wide range of color intensities and you and your colorist should work together to select a shade that fits you and your life-style. The quality of the final result depends on the combination of your colorist's talent and your own self-image. The clearer you can be in your own mind about what changes you want to make, the more successful the results are likely to be.

7 *Scalp and hair condition.* Evaluate the present physical condition of these important factors. Is your scalp dry, flaky, irritated by a rash, excessively oily? Is the hair brittle from overprocessing with chemicals, is it dull, split at the ends? I feel it's best to determine this by having a professional consultation (often given free at salons). And that holds true even if you decide to be your own colorist at home. Either way, your scalp and hair should be as healthy as possible before any coloring processing takes place.

8 *Slight graying.* If you are just beginning to gray, consider the subtle change of a rinse. Or think about adding highlights that will detract from the gray. Remember, there are many ways to alter gray other than by simply applying straight hair color.

9 *Total graying.* If your hair is very gray or totally gray, always select a shade that is lighter than your own, never darker. (See Chapter 15 for more details.)

10 *Coloring at home.* If this is your preference, be sure you are ready to do it right. Learn the procedure, preferably by watching a professional in action. Make a checklist of all the tools you need and have them on hand when you start the coloring process. There's nothing worse than being in the middle of a critical step and discovering you don't have the right equipment.

CHOOSING THE RIGHT COLOR

If you've decided that a color change is definitely what you want—and what you can deal with—you're probably ready to whiz through the color selection process. But be patient. Finding your best shade can be as difficult as locating that proverbial needle in the haystack. I have found that a sensible, educated, step-by-step approach will get you rewarding results with a minimum of agonizing over the options.

First, remember to use skin tone and eye color as your best guides to hair color. The color you choose should enhance your skin shade and brighten your eyes. A handy tip to keep in mind: Your eyebrow shade represents your natural color, so try to stay within one or two shades of that. Keep in mind, too, that the older you become, the more your natural hair color fades and turns mousy. That's when hair needs a lift the most. But whatever color you decide on, *don't ever* go back to childhood color! Chances are it won't suit you any longer, since your skin tone isn't what is used to be. It's a better idea to try one of the warmer shades that will compliment your eyes, your skin, your personality as they are now. Another mistake to avoid: Don't decide on a dramatic shade because it looks great on your favorite model or entertainer or whomever. Remember, you are the one who will have to live with the color. And you are the person the color should be compatible with.

FINDING A COLORIST

If you've already gone through the tedious trial-and-error procedure of selecting a good dentist or doctor, you'll know that once you've landed one to your liking, he or she is yours for life. Well, the same holds true for your colorist. Finding the one who's right for you can be a long and arduous task. Unfortunately, however, too many women elevate their colorists to superhuman status and think they can do no wrong or harm. Even though colorists are trained technicians, they are human; they can and will and do make mistakes. Also, you need to realize that some colorists are making major decisions every day and with less than a few minutes in which to diagnose and remedy a client's problem. Without a doubt, some colorists *are* more qualified than others. How to find them is the question. The best places have traditionally been from the pages of fashion and beauty magazines. Try writing to the beauty editors or reader service departments of these publications and they will gladly provide you with the information you request, if it is available. The second best source is from the recommendations of satisfied friends and relatives. If your stylist is also your colorist, that person should be expert enough in the coloring process to be able to answer all your questions and do the color work properly. If not, I suggest you look for a color specialist.

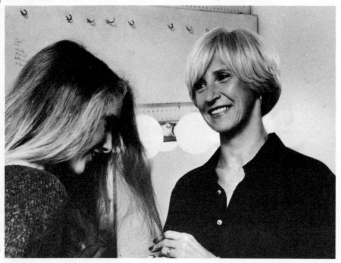

THE COLOR PROCESS

The type of color process used depends on which color direction you select or how light or dark you go. First, you should understand the difference between a single-process and a double-process application.

A double-process application means the hair is bleached, lightened, or stripped of its natural color first, after which a color tint toner is applied to produce the final color. A toner is similar in composition to any other hair colorant, but it is called a toner because its primary use is to tone down the bleached color.

The double process is used to create delicate blonde shades. To color hair this way successfully, it is necessary first to neutralize the natural color of the hair so that the applied tint can produce a better effect—making the hair a blank canvas to which you, the artist, apply the color.

The first step in this double process is to lighten or bleach the hair, and make the hair porous enough to accept and hold the tint shade. Natural color pigment is found in the cortex (middle) layer of the hair. To decolor the natural pigment, a bleaching solution—usually of ammonia and peroxide— is used. The chemicals react together to release the oxygen needed to bring about decolorization or oxidation of natural pigment. This process can lighten the hair's natural shade by as much as 2½ times.

The next step is the application of the color tint. The object here is for the tint to penetrate through the cuticle, or outer layer of the hair shaft, to the cortex, whose natural pigment has been neutralized by the lightening solution. Ammonia is a required ingredient in the formula to activate color, because the alkali in the ammonia causes the scales of the cuticle to rise, helping the tint to penetrate into the cortex.

In addition to the alkaline tint base, a developer or oxidizer—usually a 20-volume hydrogen peroxide solution—is mixed with the permanent tint color. When the molecules of the color tint base pass through the cuticle into the cortex, the color tint ingredients begin to interact with the oxidizer to join hundreds of molecules and to form into chains of color pigment molecules. These chains are too large to pass out through the cuticle scales and so are trapped within the cortex, making the tinting process a *permanent* change.

A single-process application means that the bleach (lightener) and toner (color tint) are combined in one product. This is usually the procedure used when the desired color is close to your natural hair color. Since the chemicals are applied once instead of twice, a single-process treatment is less damaging to hair.

The general rule about hair coloring is this: The farther away your desired color ranges from your natural color, the more chemicals are necessary to achieve it. Therefore, the more damaging the process is likely to be. The nearer one is to the other, the less damaging the process. For example, a dark brunette can never become blonde without using a double-process coloring because it is necessary first to lighten her natural color pigment sufficiently so that the new color will take and show effectively. This means bleaching and toning separately. But a woman with light to medium brown hair can become a dark blonde by means of a single-process tint.

Either process can be professionally applied or done at home from commercially packaged products. Single-process tints can be purchased in a variety of shades for women desiring one or two shades lighter than normal color. The easiest to use are the shampoo-in types. These eliminate retouching, since all you do is shampoo the hair again to retint it. However, even these processes contain chemicals, so be cautious with those sensitive ends. Depending on the contrast between your natural color and the applied color, growth lines will be visible within three to four weeks. So to discourage breakage, allow the full four weeks (and longer if possible) to pass before retouching. My advice: Stick to within one or two shades from your natural color for less damage and a more realistic color effect.

Retouching. This process may vary from salon to salon. And certain methods are more damaging than others. In simple color retouching, chemicals are applied only to the new growth, usually around the root areas.

When hair has been highlighted, the retouching methods can vary from the cap method to the foil system (see Chapter 13).

Whatever retouching method is used, a big part of its success is in keeping your hair in healthy condition. Regular deep conditioning is a must for treated hair. Chemicals leave hair dry and brittle, and only when you embark on a consistent conditioning regimen will you insure great color along with healthy hair (see Chapter 9).

One last tip: When retouching at home, make sure you apply the color only to the new growth. Nature is always your best example, and hair is naturally lighter at the ends, not darker. So I advise retouching when your color has faded from using other chemical processes such as permanent waving or straightening. I also recommend retouching when you have finished with a long period in the sun (either summer or winter). Constant reapplication of chemicals to already treated ends will only cause further breakage and a chronic case of the "dulls."

Home Coloring. With salon prices keeping pace with inflation, home coloring—primarily tinting and hennas—has become very popular. The simplicity of the packaged formulas leads a lot of women to experiment with various colors at home, and because most home colorists are cautious, the results are quite successful. I believe you can create just about any color process by yourself at home. All it takes is careful reading of the package instructions, the right tools, and a little patience. If you find you're not able to handle it, go back to your salon and let a professional take over. Hair color is nothing to fool with, especially when your former golden locks start turning a surprising shade of green! If you do have a hair coloring emergency, or simply want individual help, Clairol has set up a special "hot line" for you to call for instant answers. In the continental United States, call toll-free (800) 223-5800. In New York State, call collect (212) 644-2990. Phones are in service from 8:30 a.m. to 8:00 p.m. Eastern time.

Here's my list of tips for home coloring, which I devised over years of experience and seeing the results of common mistakes women make.

1. Buy everything necessary for a complete job before starting. Read the product label to see what tools are required. The usual list includes: brush, glass or plastic bowl, rat-tail comb, clips.

2. Take a patch test. Practically every commercially sold formula recommends doing this prior to application to determine whether or not you will have a normal or allergic reaction to the chemicals. Don't take this precaution lightly, for you just may be the rare person who develops contact dermatitis from the chemicals in aniline hair dyes. The patch test is simple: Mix a small amount of color according to the directions. Apply a patch of color behind the ear, on your neck, and on the inside of your arm. Let it dry com-

pletely; this usually takes about 10 minutes. Wait 24 hours and then check your skin in those areas. If it is irritated, red, or rashy, don't use the product. But this doesn't mean you have to give up hair coloring altogether. Try switching to another brand. You might be allergic to one chemical combination and not another. However, if the patch is normal, the product is safe.

3. Try a "preview test" to see how your hair will react to the color. Snip off a small strand of hair from underneath, at the back of your head. Tape it to a piece of cardboard. Apply the color according to directions. In a very short time you'll be able to see for yourself exactly how your hair will take to the color.

4. Apply the hair color starting at the crown of the head and working down to the nape. Then work on the front. This will save a lot of hair breakage in the front because chemicals won't be on as long as they are in the back.

5. Use a three-way mirror to see exactly what you are doing. Don't rely on guesswork. Retouching, especially, can be very difficult to do properly if you can't see all sides of your head.

6. Have a color party. Invite a friend or two to share the color experience. You can apply color to each other's hair. This helps eliminate many of the common mistakes, saves time, and turns a lot of worrying into a lot of laughs.

7. Follow the timing instructions to the split second. These will be clearly provided in the product directions. Classically, the biggest cause of poor home coloring is improper timing.

THE REVERSE PROCESS

If years of overbleaching have turned you into an unnaturally harsh blonde—or if you're just plain weary of the constant cost and time-consuming touch-up trips for any color—don't wait for the color to grow out (usually six months to a year of living with an unwanted color) before changing it or adding streaks. I have had excellent results in "reversing" any shade from blonde to red

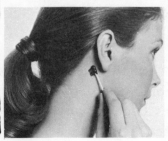
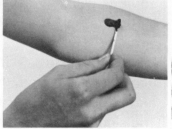

back to normal or, at least, to within one or two shades of normal. Adding streaks of any shade to light blonde hair is called **reverse sunbursting;** for dark blonde to medium brown hair, the process is called **reverse tortoiseshelling.**

I use a semipermanent color for my reverse-process treatments because I find it less damaging and more accurate than the arduous stripping of color and reapplying of another color. And even better, the entire procedure is less than one hour long, rather than the usual 6-hour nightmare. If the treatment is done properly, hair will turn out looking as if it had never been colored before.

Different colorists use different methods, and these vary according to the colorist's experience and degree of interest in keeping hair healthy. Old-fashioned processes often damaged hair considerably because chemical was placed on top of chemical and was usually washed out after two or three shampoos. The newer reverse process with semipermanent color does not fade as quickly and tends to leave hair healthier and shinier. Today's salons use either a color tint or a semipermanent color in their reverse processes. The latter creates less damage than the tint. Ask your colorist which system he or she uses.

A few color tips: A former blonde should reverse to a blonde-oriented shade rather than to a darker color for the first time. Otherwise the drastic change could be a real shocker.

In detail, here's how the reverse sunburst and tortoiseshell procedures work. Streaks are woven into the regrowth and separated from the rest of the hair. The remainder is reversed back to the shade most closely related to your natural color. To maintain the sunburst or tortoiseshell effect, reapplication is necessary every three months. To extend its life, I suggest using a mild shampoo. However, if you reversed back to your normal color, retouching will not be necessary (unless the hair is extremely damaged or porous, in which case two applications will be required for a perfect result). If a semipermanent color has been used, don't worry about the damage; there is none.

COLOR DYES AND YOUR HEALTH

The recent attempt to label certain hair dye chemicals as health hazards has stirred a hornet's nest of controversy about hair color product ingredients and human safety.

The background is as follows: In 1978 the U.S. Food and Drug Adminstration proposed a regulation that would require a warning label to appear on all dyes containing a widely used chemical, 4-MMPD. Triggering this was the National Cancer Institute's report on test results, showing that thirteen hair dye chemicals (including 4-MMPD) caused cancer in animals.

The hair color industry strongly disagrees that this ingredient poses potential risks to humans. However, they have reformulated their hair color products and have removed 4-MMPD, not because they concur with the proposed danger, but to prevent the public from unnecessary worry until the FDA's uncertainty is resolved.

Color Damage. Unfortunately, no chemical process can be done without some damage to the hair. Chemicals placed on untreated hair will do less harm than those placed on treated hair. In effect, what's happening is that chemical is being placed on chemical. This is why the retouching process must be done with great care.

You can minimize color damage by taking extra care of your hair with gentle shampooing, conditioning treatments, and avoidance of overexposure to heat and sunlight. And if you want to try a less radical color change, think of highlighting instead. That's what the next chapter is all about.

Hair color should harmonize with the color tone of your skin and the color of your eyes. Also, lip and cheek tints should not be ignored since they relate to hair and the overall look.

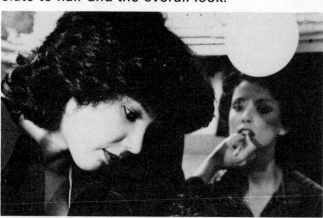

MEDIUM/MEDIUM SALLOW SKIN TONE

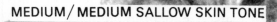

BLUE EYES		BROWN EYES		HAZEL EYES	
HAIR	CHEEKS/LIPS	HAIR	CHEEKS/LIPS	HAIR	CHEEKS/LIPS
—Pale blonde (Swedish tone) —Blonde streaks —Reddish tones (freckled skin)	—Copper —Light russet	—Blonde shades (no platinum or silver tones) —Blonde highlights —Tortoise-shell	—Amber brown —Red brown	—Peach —Strawberry —Pale blonde (Swedish tone) —Blonde streaks	—Copper —Light russet

DARK / DARK SALLOW SKIN TONE

BLUE EYES		BROWN EYES		HAZEL EYES	
HAIR	CHEEKS/LIPS	HAIR	CHEEKS/LIPS	HAIR	CHEEKS/LIPS
Keep your natural hair color	—Bright copper —Bright russet	—Natural color —Red highlights —Blonde highlights	—Red —Russet —Bordeaux —Peach —Rust —Amber —Plum	Keep your natural hair color	—Bright copper —Bright russet

LIGHT SKIN TONE

BLUE EYES		BROWN EYES		HAZEL EYES	
HAIR	CHEEKS/LIPS	HAIR	CHEEKS/LIPS	HAIR	CHEEKS/LIPS
—Beige —Golden blonde —Tawny	—Peach —Dusty rose	—Blonde highlights	—Peach —Coral —Pink —Plum	—Beige —Dark golden blonde —Tawny blonde highlights	—Peach —Dusty rose

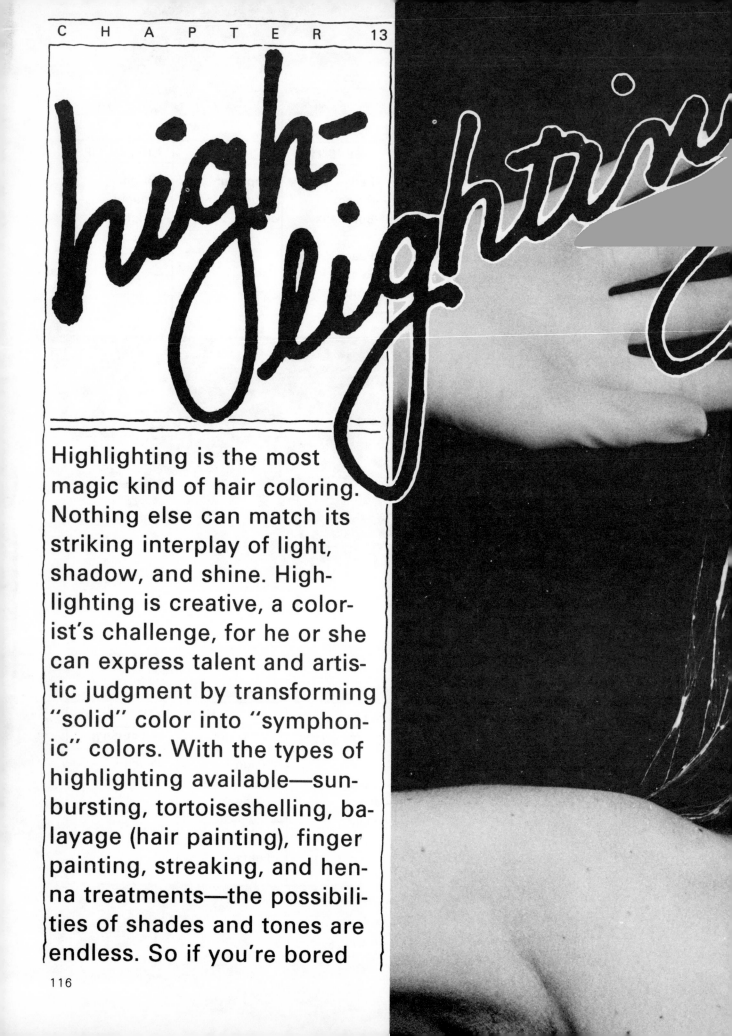

high-lighting

Highlighting is the most magic kind of hair coloring. Nothing else can match its striking interplay of light, shadow, and shine. Highlighting is creative, a colorist's challenge, for he or she can express talent and artistic judgment by transforming "solid" color into "symphonic" colors. With the types of highlighting available—sunbursting, tortoiseshelling, balayage (hair painting), finger painting, streaking, and henna treatments—the possibilities of shades and tones are endless. So if you're bored

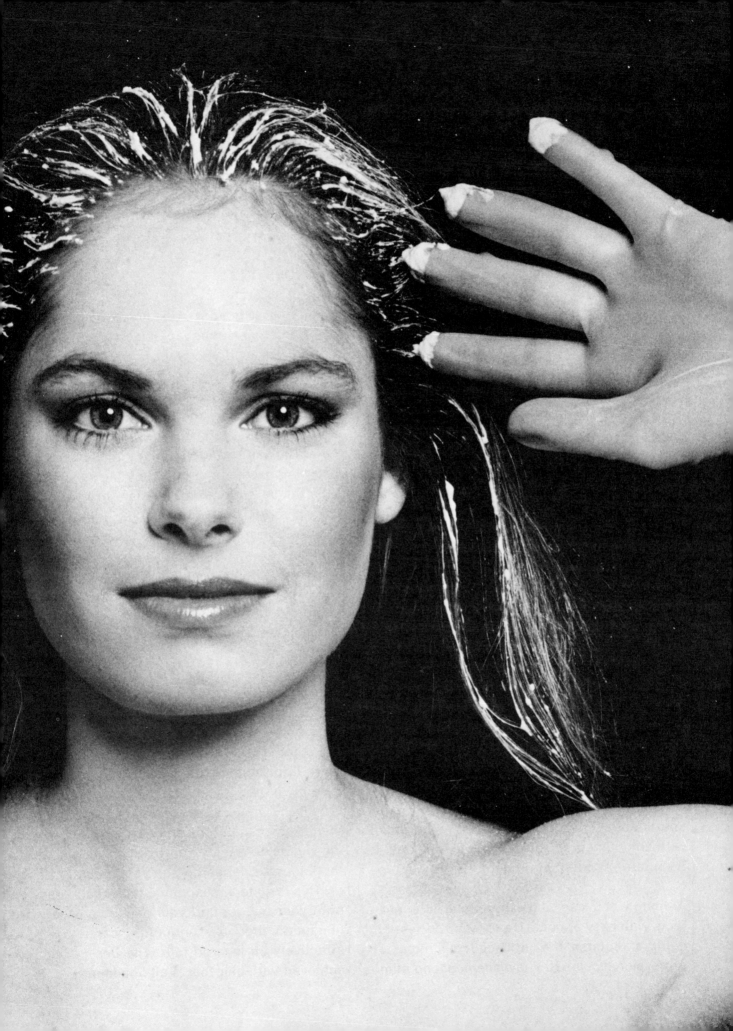

with coloring your hair all one way, try a special effect. One that's right for you. One that will become your look, your signature. There are a few "watch-for" guidelines I would like to share with you as we discuss each highlighting process. But first I want to talk about what highlighting actually is and does to hair, and to you.

Highlighting adds lighter and brighter and shinier streaks to your hair to produce a soft and natural blonde effect. Try to keep nature in mind when using this process. For example, salt-and-pepper combinations (a very contrasting mix of dark and light highlights) are not only unnatural, they're old-fashioned. They're also not very stylish and can even be misread as dark hair turning gray. Brunettes need a word of warning because they will often ask for blonde highlights, thinking these will create a dramatic and exciting look. But beware! They won't. The effect will usually be too harsh, especially on a younger woman. So I discourage the idea. Don't ask for light blonde streaks unless your hair is normally light. Streaks that are too light tend to cause a "graying" effect. If you just remember not to introduce a shade that isn't already present in your hair, you'll be safe. Your colorist should combine your natural color with complimentary shades so the total look will be subtle yet confident, bright yet not blaring.

Although you can achieve wonderful sunlit effects with easy at-home treatments, perfect highlighting requires the practiced technique of a professional colorist. The *placement and number* of streaks are the two most important factors in successful highlighting. There's no set formula for either because they depend on your hair length and the colorist's creative eye. But incorrect placement and/or overcrowding of streaks will produce an artifical look rather than the natural, normal effect you're after.

SUNBURSTING

If you want to get out of the bleached-blonde bind of having hair retouched every month, try a sunburst process. If you want to prolong those natural summer highlights all year long, again I say try sunbursting. It is the youngest looking and most natural of all the highlighting processes—and the easiest to keep up. Why? Because it imitates the natural highlighting that happens when your hair has been streaked by the sun. Hair that is in the light blonde to medium brown range is the best for these sun-kissed highlights. The streaks are made with paste bleach placed only on hair from the topmost layer, beginning at the crown and then continuing down the hair strands right to the ends. Those strands are selected by using the tip of a rat-tail comb to weave through and pick up a thin row of hair. The hairs are then wrapped in aluminum foil. When all the streaks are processed, the hair is shampooed and conditioned. The finer the streaks, the more natural the look. Because there is no specific pattern to the streaking, it results in random, more natural-looking color. The hairline and part are avoided so there is no demarcation line to worry about as monthly growth takes place. If you decide not to repeat the process, all the streaks will gradually blend with your natural color. Otherwise, retouching will be necessary approximately every two to three months depending on your natural hair color. This is quite a reasonable time span—easy on both your budget and your schedule. One word of caution, though—sunbursting cannot be done effectively on layered hair. The best results are achieved with hair that is all one length.

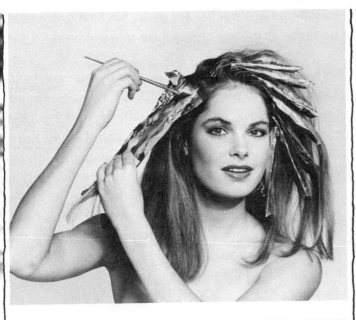

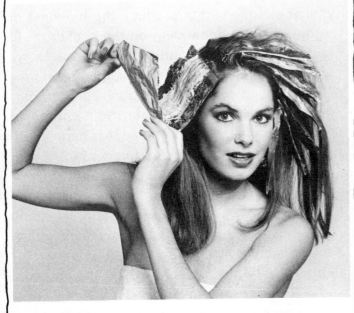

This mixed color effect produces an interesting quality that combines richness with delicacy. But remember, you have to begin with the proper shade of brown hair to achieve maximum effectiveness. As with sunbursting, hair should be all one length to look its best with tortoiseshell highlights. Another budget softener, tortoiseshelling is easy on your wallet because retouching is necessary only after two to three months.

BALAYAGE (HAIR PAINTING)

Balayage and sunbursting are practically twin methods since their application and effect vary only slightly; but though balayage has a subtlety all its own, its effect is not as bright as that of sunbursting and is seen only if done on very light hair. Like sunbursting, it involves a series of streaks (thinner than sunbursting) placed on the top of the head, without touching the hairline and usually painted away from the part rather than on it. The bleach is brushed on with an artist's brush so all the hairs are not bleached to the same degree. Only a few strands of hair are affected, which creates a natural effect—as if the sun did the highlighting and not the colorist. There are no growth lines, and streaks will gradually blend with your normal color. However, retouching can be done every four to five months if you want to keep looking fresh. Hair painting looks best on short to medium-length hair. For longer hair, sunbursting's foil method is more effective.

With balayage or with sunbursting streaks, don't worry about sitting in the sun. As long as your hair is in good condition, the sun will not hurt it—despite what conventional wisdom says about protecting all color-treated hair from the sun. Sometimes streaks and highlights look better if the sun lightens them further; and when the background shade is also sun-lightened, it creates an even more natural look than you expected. So why not undress your head? Forget about your hat and scarf. Be free! Have fun in the sun.

TORTOISESHELLING

This highlighting process derives its name from the tortoiseshell's deep red and gold tones. It is basically the same as sunbursting, but is done on medium to dark brown hair. It will add subtle, fiery tones to dull, mousy brown hair. The streaks themselves are a mixture of dark blonde and light brown tones or soft cognac and brandy shades depending on the background color of your hair. The darker the backdrop, the darker the streaks.

FINGER PAINTING

This is an easy at-home highlighting process that creates very subtle blonde effects. The best results happen when you want only a few strands of blonde in front. The at-home method is simple because the color highlights are actually rubbed through your hair with your fingers. The motion is the same as brushing hair away from your face with your fingers. It's an ideal answer for people who don't like to subject their hair to the foil paper, cap, or weaving methods.

When doing your own at-home process it is necessary to wear a pair of thin plastic gloves. Prepare the "finger paint" carefully, according to the exact directions. Dip four gloved fingers into the bleach solution. Then run your fingers through your hair as if your were pushing it back off your face, starting at the front hairline and working back to whatever point you want to stop. Leave the solution on for the time specified on the package label. Then rinse off, shampoo, and condition. You'll love the instant "blonding" results.

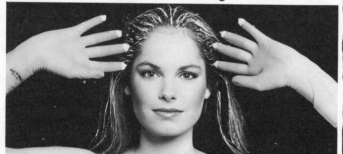

STREAKING

Half-head Streaking. This highlighting process—like whole-head streaking (below)—produces a brighter and lighter effect because highlights are placed at the sides and crown from ear to ear. The technique is like that used in sunbursting: The colorist selects strands of hair with a rat-tail comb, applies paste bleach to them, and wraps them in foil. Half-head highlights should be placed close to the hairline for best results and to attract more brightness to your face. However, touch-ups are necessary every six to eight weeks because growth lines will be more visible.

Whole-head Streaking. With this process, highlights are placed throughout the *entire* head, underneath and close to the hairline, making it the most expensive and time-consuming of all lightening techniques. Women with hair all one length do have an advantage here: They needn't bother with streaking the layers underneath because they are rarely seen (unless you wear your hair up). Women with layered haircuts must highlight the entire head because unless all the different lengths are lightened, the effect is unfinished and certainly not as dramatic as it could be.

Whole-head highlights produce the blondest or brightest effect, depending on the backdrop. To create this degree of lightness, many streaks are placed close to the hairline and hair part, with the resulting need for frequent touch-ups, approximately every six to eight weeks. So be prepared to spend about 1½ hours and approximately $60 to $75 per visit when you go this route.

After months of retouching, hair damage and breakage are inevitable. The constant bleaching of the most sensitive portions of the hair (hairline and top area) makes them weak and vulnerable to breakage. On short, layered cuts the ends will suffer from repeated overbleaching. This can be controlled somewhat more easily because short hairs are trimmed frequently and damaged parts are usually snipped off in the process. Another concern is that the colorist cannot pick out the exact streaks bleached before, since hairs blend together so closely. He or she *could* spend hours and hours searching—at what cost—and might be able to avoid some of the problem of rebleaching the same hairs. But that usually isn't the case, and so you may find yourself going blonder in certain areas than you like. If this happens, try a reverse sunburst process (see Chapter 12) once a year to control the amount of blonde buildup.

Do-it-yourself Streaking. Home streaking can be done with great success and ease if you use the correct method, the right tools, and follow label instructions very carefully. There are, to be sure, risks involved: Hair breakage from overprocessing is one risk; ending up with the wrong shade is another, because not all hair takes color the same way. But the benefits are time and money saved, and individual control over the results you get. Also, a patch test isn't necessary with this streaking process because chemicals don't come into contact with the scalp or skin. I recommend against using kits that rely on the perforated cap method, which directs you to place the cap on your head and pull the hair strands through the holes. This system may be easy, but it's like working in the dark. There is no way to see exactly where the highlights are placed. It's a guessing game all the way—with the odds against good results. I prefer using the foil method described below, which insures a more professional finish and gives you total control over how many streaks you want and where you want them.

Before you begin, it's very important to realize that this kind of streaking is more flattering on medium brown to light brown hair. But whatever your background color, always do streaking on dry hair. That said, here are step-by-step instructions for how to proceed.

· · · · · · · · ·T·O·O·L·S· · · · · · · · ·
You don't need very much: a streaking kit, toothbrush, foil, a nonmetal bowl for the bleach, rat-tail comb, and hair clips.

· · · ·T·E·C·H·N·I·Q·U·E·S· · · · ·
1. Hold back the hairline hair with clips ¼" deep around the face so you won't streak it. This avoids an obvious line next to your face when streaks begin to grow out. If you wear a part, start streaks just below the part.
2. Cut about 12 pieces of foil, each 4" wide by 6" long.

3. Mix bleach paste according to kit directions. Make sure it's not too thick to start with; it will thicken by itself as you use it.
4. Using the tip of the rat-tail comb, pick up in a weaving motion a thin row of hair starting on the top of your head. Don't take up too much. Be sure you're working horizontally. Don't go any farther toward the back of your head than you can see easily or reach with the tail length of the comb.
5. Pick up a sheet of foil. Fold back one edge of it about 2" to give you a thick edge like a hem. Push this under the hair you've picked up.
6. Load the toothbrush with bleach paste.
7. Using the brush, cover the row of woven hairs with bleach.
8. Fold the bottom of the foil up over the hair ends. Fold again so the edges meet at the scalp. Fold sides toward the center to seal completely.
9. Now you're ready to do your next row, which should be about ½" below the first. Rows should be spaced about ½" apart. Clip hair that you are not streaking to the foil above it.
10. Take another row and repeat the bleaching and foil-wrapping steps. Continue this way until you reach the end of your hair.
11. After you finish wrapping your hair, go back and check the color of the very first streaks you did. Remove the foil. Scrape a bit of bleach off with your finger so you can see the hair. All the red and orangey tones should be gone. Hair should look a pale golden blonde. If it still looks orangey, apply more bleach and close up foil. Check for color again in 5 minutes.
12. You'll take the first streaks down before the last since they've had a longer time to be processed. As streaks reach the color you want, rinse them individually with a cup of warm water to remove bleach.
13. When all streaks are processed, shampoo and condition your hair. You'll love the results—even better, the fact that you did it all yourself. And just count up all the money you saved! So why not treat yourself to something very special? You deserve it.

HENNA

The subject of highlighting would not be complete without discussing henna, which has come into vogue in the last few years along with all kinds of other "retro" fashions. Henna dates back to ancient Egyptian times, when Cleopatra used it. Many modern-day beauties have also chosen this method, but despite its popularity through the centuries, its performance rating is poor and it is a technique I hesitate to recommend.

The last widespread rage for red-hued hair was in the late 1930s, when the label "carrot top" came into use for hennaed redheads. What henna did then, and still does, is to turn hair into some of the strangest orangey-red colors imaginable—great for sunsets, but not for hair. Alas, the fad returned in the late 1970s. Because it's a "natural" coloring agent, it seemed the logical non-chemical alternative to hair coloring for many ecology-minded, back-to-earth beauties.

It's true that henna is a natural product, derived from the cut, dried, and powdered leaves—and, in some cases, the stalks—of the plant *Lawsonia inermis.* The powder, which has a greenish-gray cast to it, is mixed with hot water to release the henna color—red. To color or highlight your hair with henna, you apply the paste mixture and leave it on for one hour. This "natural" process has its drawbacks. Henna is gritty to feel, has a rather strong and unpleasant odor, and can leave an unpredictable color palette—anything from subtle red highlights on untreated hair to an interesting shade of green on permed hair.

What Is Pure Henna? Pure henna is what most people think of when they ask for a henna treatment—the derivative of the *leaves* of the henna plant. Nothing else is added. Pure henna gives you a red color—no more, no less. When applied to different shades of hair, it will achieve different effects:

- •*on dark brown-black hair* there is hardly a visible take. Some red highlights might come through if you leave the henna paste on for at least one hour.
- •*on light brown hair,* the ideal shade for henna, you see the transition and red highlights easily.
- •*on blondish hair* henna tends to get orangey.
- •*on gray hair* it goes even more orangey—giving you a look that's somewhere between Howdy Doody and Raggedy Ann. Fine for make-believe folk, but not so fashionable on mature women!

What Is Compound Henna? It is pure henna mixed with metallic salts to produce colors other than red. The variety of color options it offers is the reason for its popularity; but, as its name implies, compound henna can compound the problems of pure henna. In addition to possible discoloration, it will also cause hair to break off if hair undergoes chemical treatments such as permanent waving or straightening. Until recently, many beauty salons didn't understand the complications of this seemingly innocent "natural" product, and as a result proceeded to wipe a lot of locks off pretty heads.

Henna and herbs. When metallic salts are not added to pure henna, herbs are used for the same purpose—to create colors other than red. Indigo is one such popular herb, used for centuries in the textile industry to dye fabrics a blue color. Chestnuts and walnuts are used to give brown shades. The list of additives could go on and on; and all of them are usually snapped up by the unknowing and trusting consumer who loves the reassuring sound of anything magical and "natural" at the same time.

What Is Neutral Henna? Actually it's not henna at all, strictly speaking. It's made from the stalks and stems of the henna plant rather than from the leaves, and there is absolutely no color in these parts. So neutral henna will not give you *any* color highlights. It can, however, add body to your hair.

Henna Is Forever. Once henna is on the hair, there is no way to remove it (except with one very special Clairol product called Metallex). And if you should decide after a while that you're tired of your henna highlights, you'll have to wait for them to grow out, or cut them off—or live with them. Even though most people think henna simply coats the hair, in fact it actually penetrates into the cuticle, which is the protective outermost layer of the hair. Henna's gritty texture can damage the cuticle, and this can lead to injury of the cortex—the largest, most important layer of the hair, which is responsible for strength, elasticity, and pliability.

While you're living with your hennaed hair there are lots of treatments that become taboo. Permanent waving, chemical straightening, coloring, tinting, or highlighting can all cause problems. Obviously, this limits your options, so if you insist on henna you must have a strategy for your hair for at least six months to come.

For example, if you want to have your hair straightened or permed and you already have henna in it, you should wait six months before doing so. Keep your hair in shape with a good haircut during those months; then, when the henna has had a chance to grow out, you can perm or straighten your hair safely. The same is true for color. You cannot apply henna on color or color on henna in rotation. *Either* you apply color on henna *or* henna on color; if you want to switch completely from one to the other, give your hair a rest of six months. Hair just cannot take that much abuse without serious damage.

Henna and Other Coloring Processes. If your hair is colored anywhere from light brown to any of the darker shades, you can apply henna on top of the color treatment as long as the henna is in the same shade as your other color. If you have henna to start with and want to add color, you can do so—as long as the hair color is the same shade as the henna. Don't try to go lighter. If you try to add color highlights to hair that is already hennaed, the henna will make the highlight turn a strange green shade ... which, by the way, is nearly impossible to remove from the hair. If you decide to have your untreated hair streaked first and then hennaed, there is an effective procedure. Have the hair streaked and bleached out to a golden level and *then* apply the henna color. Henna applied on streaked hair will not wash out because bleach creates porosity and the henna then has something to "grab" on to. You'll have streaks or highlights of a hennaed red, or of whatever shade the kind of henna you've chosen produces.

Henna and Permanent Waving. Combine them in a certain sequence and you'll have a titanic disaster on your hands ... and head! If your hair has been hennaed first, the chemicals in a perm solution will react with the henna and discolor your hair badly. It will usually go brownish to greenish. Henna also interferes with the effectiveness of the perm's curl because it won't allow the hair to absorb the lotion as well. However, if you have a permanent wave first and then a henna treatment, the results will be satisfactory. But it's important to remember that it only works with *one* henna application. The second go-round with henna will be bad news. Unless, of course, you decide against another perm. If you do, I recommend you use henna a maximum of three times a year—no more. If you're letting the henna grow out, keep cutting your hair at frequent intervals and the transition stage will be less noticeable.

Henna and Chemical Straightening. The same problems apply to using henna first and straighteners second, except that if you do, chances are that the discoloration will be even more extreme. But if you reverse the procedures, with a relaxer first and henna afterward, you should have no trouble.

Henna—What Else It Does. Now that I've run down the long list of henna misuses, let me tell you a few of its other functions. If you use it carefully and sensibly henna can do more than just color your hair.

Henna and oiliness. Henna has a drying effect on the scalp, and so it is one way of controlling an oily condition. Buy why bother when there are so many other easier, healthier, and more effective methods available to do the job?

Henna and shine. Yes, it'll give extra shine . . . the first time you use it. But repeated applications will cause a buildup that coats the hair and gives you a very unhappy case of dullness. I recommend you stick to no more than three henna applications a year.

Henna and body. Neutral henna, when applied to the hair, will coat the hair shafts and give them bulk and body. However, if you don't rinse it out well, the gritty residue can be abrasive and damaging to the hair. And if you rinse it away completely, you negate the whole purpose of putting it on in the first place! So if you're using henna to give your hair body, treat it with extra care afterward.

Henna and red highlights. If that's all you want, henna away . . . especially if you have light or medium brown hair. To get great-looking red highlights, apply the henna to hair that's all one length, the same way you would with sunbursting. The highlights won't rinse out with this system, and you can retouch them on the new growth just as you would with any other retouching process. And since you're only applying it to a few strands of hair, damage is kept to a minimum. But always apply a conditioner after shampooing and treat yourself to a deep treatment once a month. It's very important to keep hair in the best shape possible if you plan on giving it *any* process treatment—even "natural" henna.

DO-IT-YOURSELF COLORED HENNA

· · · · · · · · T·O·O·L·S · · · · · · · · ·
henna powder
Vaseline
rubber gloves
brush and comb
mixing dish
plastic bag or foil
cotton

· · · · · T·E·C·H·N·I·Q·U·E · · · · ·
1. Buy henna powder in a drug, health, or beauty supply store.
2. Mix 6 ounces of henna with 6 ounces of hot tap water to form a paste the consistency of thick shampoo. Follow instructions carefully. Let stand 2 to 3 minutes for extra thickening.
3. Apply Vaseline to hairline, ears, and neck. This prevents discoloration of the skin.
4. Always protect your hands with rubber gloves.
5. Apply the henna to clean, dry hair. If the hair is extremely soiled, shampoo it lightly and towel-dry it first.
6. Section the hair and start at the crown area, applying the henna with a brush from roots to ends. Cover the entire head with henna and comb through hair to distribute evenly.
7. Wrap head with a plastic bag or kitchen foil. Place a coil of cotton around the hairline to prevent dripping.
8. Sit under a dryer 30 to 60 minutes, depending on the desired color. Check label directions.
9. Rinse thoroughly with warm water. Shampoo as usual with an acid-balanced shampoo. Follow with a cold rinse and dry as usual. Be sure to use an old towel or henna will stain more than your hair!

If—knowing that a henna treatment will lock you in and eliminate lots of other hair possibilities—you *still* want to go ahead with it, follow these

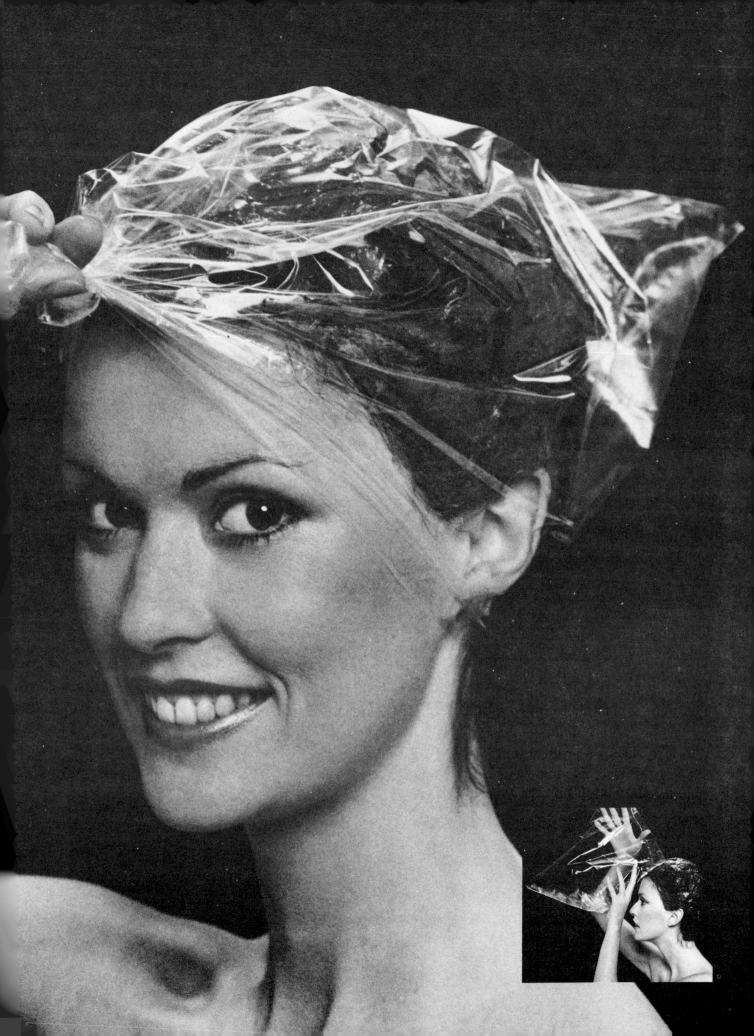

directions for the best results:

DO-IT-YOURSELF FOR NEUTRAL HENNA

· · · · · T·E·C·H·N·I·Q·U·E · · · · ·
1. Wet hair.
2. Section and apply henna with a brush from roots to ends.
3. Cover head with a plastic bag.
4. Check time (usually under 30 minutes).
5. Rinse hair extremely well with warm water.
6. Shampoo with balanced shampoo. Follow with cold rinse.

HENNA STREAKING

Streaking with henna (whether done professionally or at home) is fun and easy. Red henna produces auburn highlights on dark hair, while burgundy henna adds wine tones to an otherwise drab brunette. Henna can be tricky, so I recommend a professional job. But if you feel confident, follow the directions below.

· · · · · · · T·O·O·L·S · · · · · · · ·
100 percent natural henna
toothbrush
1 dozen 4" by 6" aluminum foil pieces
rat-tail comb
hair clips

· · · · · T·E·C·H·N·I·Q·U·E · · · · ·
1. Mix 3 ounces of henna with 3 ounces of hot tap water as directed, but try to keep the mixture the consistency of paste.
2. Take all the precautions stated in the product directions.
3. Follow the directions for home streaking and apply on clean, dry hair.
4. The entire process should take approximately 30 minutes.
5. Rinse thoroughly and shampoo with an acid-balanced shampoo. Follow with a cold rinse.

NATURAL HIGHLIGHTERS

We've run through a long list of hair highlighting processes, starting with streaking and winding up with henna. All involved ingredients (some chemical) geared to created specific highlight effects. Now I'd like to talk about some of my favorites ... "natural highlighters" that use some of nature's solutions to create great results and make the most of what you've got.

FOR DARK AND AUBURN HAIR

BLACKBERRY COCKTAIL.
Mix 6 ounces grape juice, 2 ounces medical peroxide (10-volume), and 2 ounces shampoo. Leave on hair 5 to 10 minutes. Shampoo and rinse.

HENNA ESPRESSO.
Mix 6 ounces red henna with juice of 1 lemon, 1 whole egg, ½ cup espresso coffee. Blend well. Leave on hair 10 minutes. Shampoo, rinse, and condition.

FOR LIGHT HAIR

BEACH BOY COLOR
Adds beautiful blonde highlights to light hair. Mix equal parts of sea salt with shampoo and medical peroxide (20-volume). Lather into wet hair and leave on 10 minutes. Rinse well. Shampoo hair and use a conditioner.

HENNA FLASH
Neutral henna lightens slightly while it adds body and shine. Mix 6 ounces neutral henna with 2 ounces medical peroxide (10-volume), 1 egg yolk, juice from 1 lemon. Blend well. Leave on 10 minutes. Shampoo and rinse.

COLOR WHIP
Mix equal parts of shampoo with 20-volume peroxide. Lather into wet hair leave on 5 minutes. Rinse and condition.

LEMON AND LIME SWIZZLE
Mix juice of 1 lemon and 2 limes with 1 ounce mild shampoo. Leave on 15 to 20 minutes while under the dryer or in the sun.

LEMON SQUEEZE
Squeeze 1 fresh lemon directly onto hair. Comb through. Sit in sun or under dryer. Rinse; shampoo.

FOR LIGHT TO MEDIUM BROWN HAIR

AVOCADO LIGHTENER
Gently brightens the hair while its natural oils counteract any dryness. Mix ½ ounce avocado oil with 2 ounces medical peroxide (10-volume). Leave on 10 minutes. Shampoo.

HERBAL PACK
Mix 1 tablespoon nettle, 1 tablespoon rosemary, 3 tablespoons aloe vera gel, and ½ ounce medical peroxide (10-volume). Leave on 10 minutes. Shampoo.

HENNA STREAK
Apply with paintbrush for highlighting. Mix 6 ounces red henna with 2 ounces medical peroxide (10-volume). Leave on 10 minutes.

FOR LIGHT OR RED HAIR

SUN GLOW
Boil 1 tablespoon rosemary in 1 quart of water. Add 1 tablespoon boric acid and 1 tablespoon apple cider vinegar. Strain and cool. Use as rinse after shampoo.

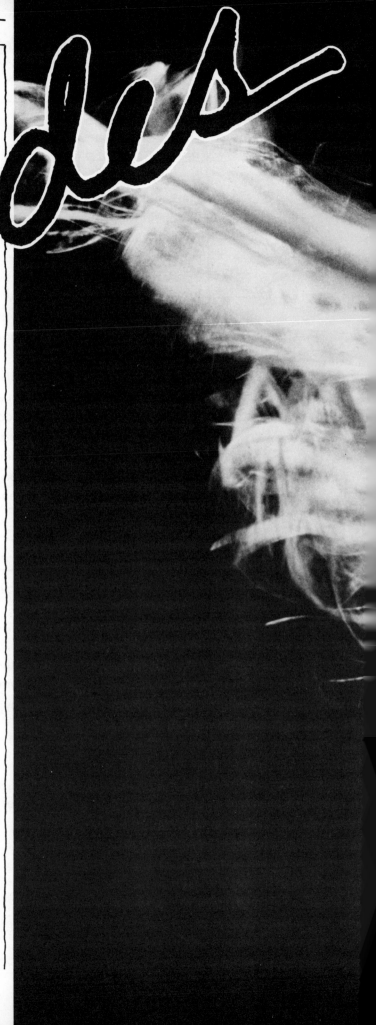

blondes

Platinum blondes like Monroe, Harlow, or Gabor might have been big box-office draws a few years back, but today that blaring, overbleached look has been packed away in the memory box. The Hollywood "egg-white" blonde with all its brash impact has been replaced—blondes now are honey-toned, warmer, more natural, subtler. And the processes by which you achieve that honey glow are gentler. Yet despite all these improvements, staying blonde is still difficult, and can be damaging.

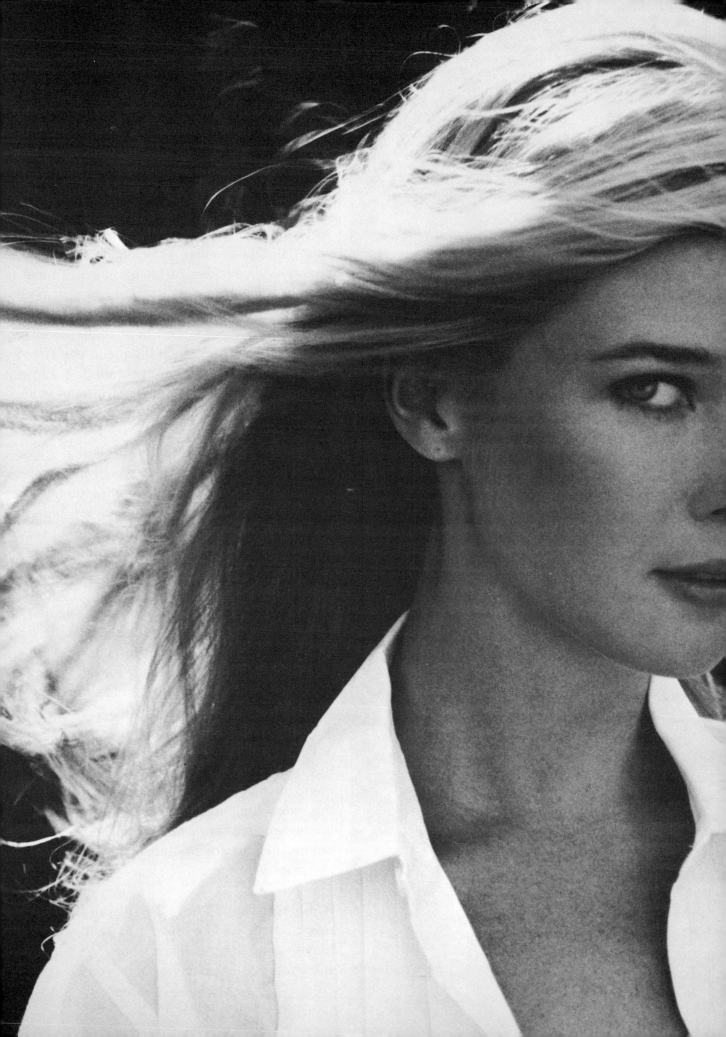

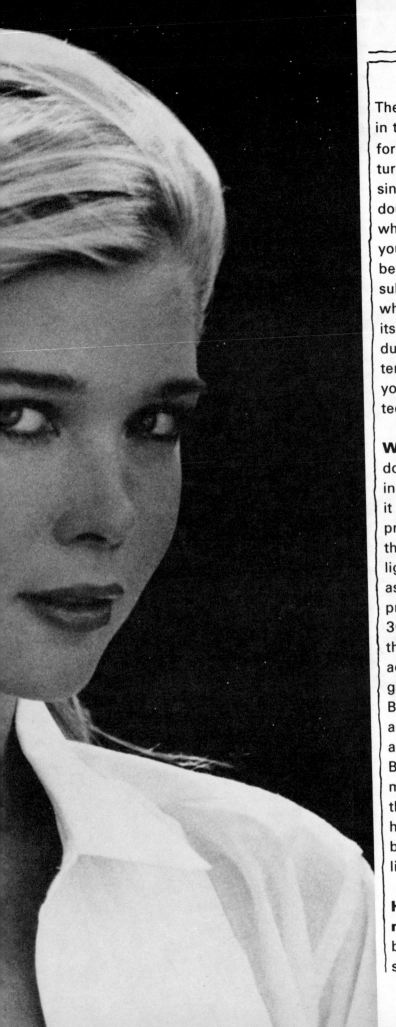

The pros and cons as well as the specific steps in the lightening process are much the same as for coloring, and for a description I suggest you turn to Chapter 12. There I mentioned that single-process coloring is less damaging than a double-process action. But it is only effective when the blonde color you're after is close to your natural hair color. That means a dark-haired beauty who decides to go blonde will have to subject her hair to a tedious double processing, which involves bleaching or stripping the hair of its natural color first and then toning it to produce the desired shade of blonde. If you are contemplating double-process coloring, I suggest you at least use what I call a "natural blonding" technique instead.

What's Natural Blonding? Essentially it is a double-processing action in which the processing time has been cut down to a fraction of what it used to be years ago. In the natural blonding process I use, the hair is prelightened *only* within the boundaries of its pigment and condition. Prelightening does not strip the hair of its pigment as much as the old system did. For example, a prelightener is applied to medium brown hair for 30 to 45 minutes. The shade that results from the bleach-out is the basis for the color to be added. Medium brown usually bleaches out to a golden blonde, while dark blonde turns flaxen. Because natural blonding minimizes the long and damaging color-stripping process, it is more advisable for the long-term health of your hair. But because it is a delicate operation, I recommend that you have a professional colorist do this work and that you don't try it yourself at home—no matter what promises of instant blonde beauty are printed on the back of hair lightener packages.

How to Keep That Born-blonde Brightness. There are lots of ways to keep your born-blonde-but-getting-darker hair on the light, bright side. You can use chemicals, or you can rely on nature. I prefer the latter way for obvious reasons, but if you want a more radical lightening and brightening than nature can give you, and you insist on chemical treatments, take heed. The easiest one-process tints are the shampoo-in variety, which eliminates retouching since all you need to do is shampoo them in again when new growth comes in. But I suggest you limit yourself to two or three reapplications; constant use of the chemicals drys out your hair and gives it an unpleasant, gummy coating. My advice is to apply the shampoo-in color *only to new growth.* This will help reduce damage and in general give your hair a more natural look.

Of course, the easiest and safest ways I know of to perk up faded blonde hair are with some of nature's best lighteners. After all, nature made the highlights die down—let it restore them! I created a few simple recipes that do just that.

Lemon and Lime Swizzle. I briefly mentioned this as a "natural highlighter" in the previous chapter. This simple recipe gives color-treated hair a rest from chemicals, while it also lightens untreated hair with absolutely no damage. So here it is again, in more detail. Blend:

> juice of 1 lemon
> juice of 2 limes
> 1 ounce of mild shampoo.

The addition of the shampoo gives the mixture body and substance so it won't drip down your face when applied. After whipping the mixture together in a bowl or blender, apply the citrusy blend to *dry hair* with a wide-toothed comb. Then sit under the dryer for 15 to 20 minutes. If you happen to be at the beach or out on your patio, apply the swizzle and then let the sun do the drying naturally. When the "setting" time is up, shampoo hair, apply a good conditioner, and you'll have instant natural highlights with no damage to your hair at all. Repeat the application in 24 hours if you want a lighter effect.

Color Whip. Another natural brightener that blondes will love is my Color Whip, also mentioned briefly in the previous chapter. Even medium brown hair can get some highlight benefits from this amazing 5-minute procedure. To repeat, blend:

> 2 ounces of mild shampoo
> 2 ounces of 20-volume peroxide.

I like to whip the ingredients together in a blender for best results. Apply the mixture to ends of hair first, working up toward the crown. Cover the hair with a "cap" of shampoo lather. Leave it on the hair for 5 minutes. Rinse thoroughly and condition. The effect is a shinier, glossier look with lots of subtle blonde highlights. The Color Whip recipe is safe for all types of hair, but I suggest that it not be overdone or you may find yourself with a grow-out problem. Once every three or four months is sufficient.

If You Want to Un-blonde. To accomplish this—or if you want to switch to another shade or go back to your natural color—I suggest you use a semipermanent rinse. This will cover up what you don't like and also let the hair that's growing in look less obviously blonde.

BRUSH-ON BLONDING

The "brush-on blonde" technique was created by me for women who prefer some fine strands of hair to be different shades of blonde (from light blonde to darker blonde) depending, of course, on the hair color they have to start with.

Brush-on blonding has many more advantages than other lightening techniques. First, it looks extremely natural, with an effect similar to what wind and sun would do to the hair. Next, the technique eliminates completely any demarcation line from grow-out, so touch-ups are not necessary. Brush-on blonding has no harsh effect on the hair. In fact, it will keep your hair looking very shiny and healthy. It will also surround your

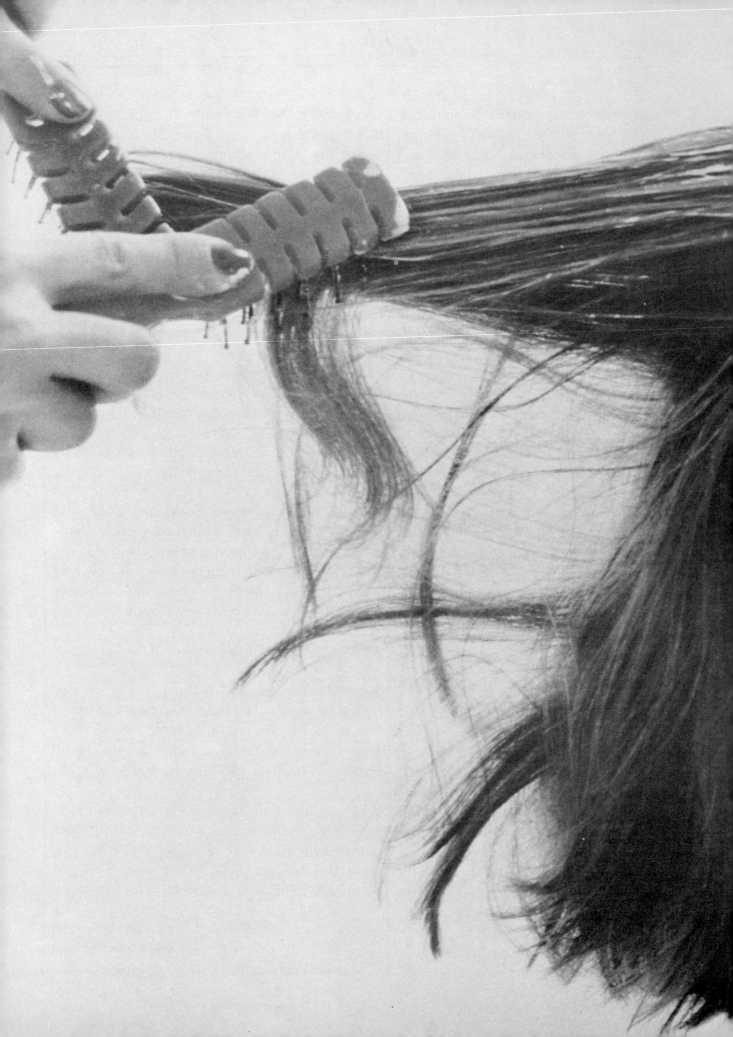

face with a new brightness and softness. And it's fabulously simple to do.

Brush-on blonding will take on any basic hair shade from light blonde to medium brown. No patch test is needed, because the chemicals never come in contact with the scalp.

· · · · · · · · · T·O·O·L·S · · · · · · · ·

Two brushes are used simultaneously during the process. One brush sections and holds hair in place so you can easily see where and what hairs to blonde. This can be any type of brush that you find comfortable to use. The second brush, used to apply the solution, is a special, small "air" or "vent" brush with 7 rows of bristles. It is available in stores and comes in lots of fun colors.

Bleaching solution: Mix 4 ounces of powdered bleach with approximately 1 ounce of 20-volume peroxide or enough to make a light paste.

1 Application of the solution is done only on the top hair area (no matter where you want the blonding to be).

2 Take a section of hair and with one downward stroke brush the bleach onto the hair, never touching the scalp.

3 Continue with all sections you want blonded. This procedure should take no more than 2 to 3 minutes.

4 Leave the blonding solution on for 5 to 10 minutes, depending on how dark your hair is to begin with.

5 Rinse off. Shampoo and condition hair.

6 If you want more blonding at a later date, you can do another brush-on blonde application in three to four months.

Blondes Need Special Care. A beautiful blonde can be a real headturner—which is probably why so many beauty magazines try for that look on their covers. As you've seen, becoming blonde is easy. Staying that way isn't. So if blonde is where you are and where you'd like to stay, take extra special care to keep your most precious asset healthy. This means special attention to shampooing and conditioning treatments. Because of the constant bleaching and retouching necessary to keep blondes at their best, their hair is prone to loss of natural moisture and flexibility. Therefore, the type of shampoo blondes use as well as the conditioners they apply should be specially formulated. I have developed two effective vitamin E-based blends that answer both needs. I strongly believe in vitamin E for *all* types of hair textures and colors because I have seen it dramatically revitalize scaling scalps and damaged hair. It also adds shine and body. My formulas are easy, do-it-yourself mixtures:

Blonde-E shampoo. Mix the contents of 1 400-unit capsule of vitamin E with 1 ounce of mild shampoo. Massage into wet hair and scalp for 3 minutes. Rinse well and finish with a cold water splash for extra shine.

Blonde-E treatment. Mix the contents of 1 400-unit capsule of vitamin E with 1 ounce of soybean oil. With a piece of cotton, apply the rich mixture lightly to the ends and wherever else the hair is most damaged. Comb through with a wide-toothed comb to distribute oils evenly. Sit under a dryer or heat cap for 15 minutes. Shampoo thoroughly by applying shampoo directly to the hair without first using water. Rinse. Then give another soaping. Finish with a cold water rinse for shine. If you've lightened your hair, I suggest deep conditioning every two weeks.

Yes, blonde hair *is* beautiful. But if you want to keep your "golden asset" going, always take the extra time and care it needs . . . and deserves!

gray hair

What to do about gray hair is a question that generates as much fuss as the subject of politics. Cover it up, leave it alone, tint it, darken it, even it out, lighten it—the directives go on and on and well-intentioned advice often causes confusion. But in the end, the best and only answer is to do what you feel is right and comfortable for *you.* If you're happy being gray, stay that way! But if you're not, know that there are lots of options available to help you turn around that inevitable sign of aging.

134

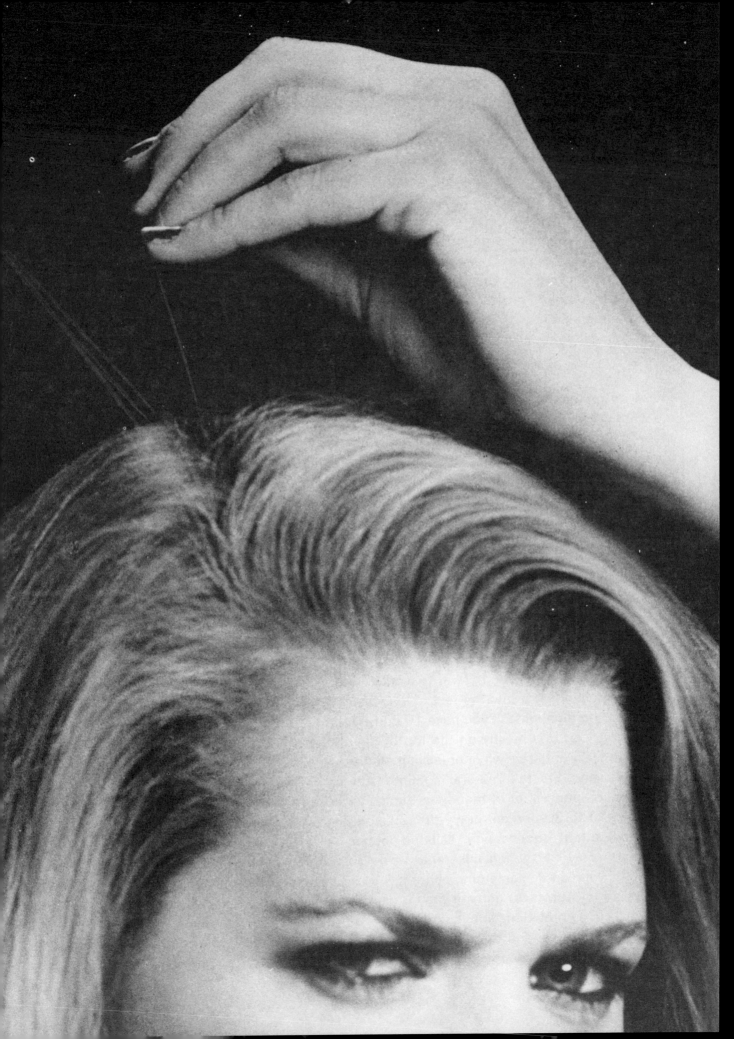

The Psychological Side. There is no doubt that gray hair is symbolic of a "mature," "responsible," or, less flattering,"middle-aged" person. But we can take some comfort in the fact that graying is the one great equalizer: Nobody escapes the graying process.

Normal graying of hair is the result of the breakdown of pigment production: as the hair root ages, color granules continue to be formed, but they are lacking in pigment. This process almost never happens overnight, and some of us go through all kinds of variations in the salt-and-pepper stage, some of them less attractive than others.

When to do what. Many times my clients ask me what I think of their gray hair—would I advise them to "do something" with it? My philosophy about gray hair is simple: No matter what percentage of gray you have, if you're not happy with it, change it. And if it doesn't bother you—if, on the contrary, you *like* it—don't change it. However, this doesn't mean you'll always feel the same way. Moods change. You change. You might want to wait until you go grayer, for example, before you make a switch. But remember that no matter what you feel, gray hair does have a tendency to make you look older.

Covering gray hair with a rinse or a tint is not the only choice or only answer. I prefer to work with the gray by blending it into the rest of your hair and by adding highlights. If you have 10 percent or less gray and it is mostly on the top of your head or in the front area, why not leave it alone? It can be a very attractive "natural highlight," the kind women spend a lot of money to duplicate. If you are 20 to 30 percent gray—that unavoidable and often unbecoming salt-and-pepper stage—you may be feeling miserable with the look. If so, you can do something about it. If your hair is 80 to 100 percent gray it can be very attractive, providing you coordinate your clothes, accessories, and makeup to blend with it. But if you're not content with that much gray,

you should know about **color wrapping,** a special process created for me by my hair coloring director, Constance Hartnett.

COLOR WRAPPING

The color-wrap process was developed as a great alternative for graying brunettes, faded redheads, and dark-haired women in general who have lost their natural rich color and want another option to all-over color, blonde streaking, or lighter highlighting. The color-wrap system mixes your own natural darker tones with richer highlights the way streaking does. Graying hair is kissed with a color close to its natural shade (instead of with a lightener), and because the gray hairs take the color differently from the nongray hairs, a marvelously complex blend of colors results, with the existing darker hairs becoming richer and the graying hairs taking on a somewhat lighter, golden glow. This "high-low" color effect is not only very natural looking, but very beautiful.

Color wrapping is really artist's work, and should be done by an experienced colorist. He or she paints a few strands with up to three tints (two is more common) that are close to your natural color, and then wraps the strands in foil. The entire procedure is fast, taking less than one hour. And it's possible to go ten to twelve weeks before retouching because new growth is more camouflaged in the interplay of colors and therefore less noticeable.

Color Tints. If your hair is over 30 percent gray, one-process tints can cover most but not all of it. If your hair is extremely gray (over 60 percent) and you're unhappy with it, turn to a more dramatic shade. But remember to keep it lighter than your own basic color, never darker. Blending the gray with your own color appears more natural. Trying to hide it will result in color that's too dark and heavy. And because of the resulting contrast, all new hair growth will be very obvious. That means more and more retouching. And more and more hair damage.

Semipermanent Color. If your gray doesn't exceed 30 percent, then it isn't necessary to use damaging tints. Try a semipermanent color product, sometimes referred to as a long-lasting rinse. It can produce natural-looking coverage without the harmful effects of a tint. It'll also give you a chance to experiment with different colors because it isn't permanent.

For fine hair, semipermanent color will cover the gray only if the gray does not exceed 30 to 40 percent. For coarse hair, it will cover gray completely if the gray doesn't exceed 20 to 25 percent. The small amount of remaining gray that will not hold the color will resemble natural highlights. And this can be a very appealing look.

Most semipermanent color lasts five to six weeks, or about eight washings, before your hair gradually fades back to its original color.

On fine hair, this type of color treatment can last up to seven or eight weeks, especially after repeated use. Since what you are applying is concentrated color, the hair will tend to collect that color after constant touch-ups. So after a time you should use the product as if it were a regular tint. Apply it first on the roots and shaft for approximately 25 minutes. Leave the ends alone; otherwise they will become coated with excess color and turn dull.

These semipermanent color products are sold in a variety of shades from blonde to black. Be very careful in picking a hair color, because what you see is not always what you get. For best results, select a color that is one shade lighter than your basic color and remember that the end result will tend to be a bit heavier and darker than what the package describes or shows.

Unfortunately, the best semipermanent color products around are sold in only a few local drug-cosmetic stores. The best sources are beauty supply stores catering to salons and other professionals—and you can find these by checking your telephone directory.

STAYING GRAY

So far I've listed all the options you can pursue if you don't want to live with your gray hair—but what if you *do*? There's no law that says that you have to pretend your hair hasn't gone gray. Besides, you may feel you like a silver-haired look. If you want to stay gray but aren't happy with the shade of gray you've turned, you can try using a shampoo-to-shampoo rinse (Roux Fanciful) or a semipermanent color (Clairol's Silk & Silver or Revlon's Glisn). These will eliminate any yellowing of gray hair without changing the rest of the color. They'll also give a beautiful gloss to hair.

Caring for Gray Hair. Though gray hair actually has a different texture than nongray hair—it's more wiry and less flexible—it doesn't need any extra care. Just use a mild shampoo and remember to condition it often and treat it to a deep treatment every now and then (see Chapter 9).

Gray Hair and Great Style. Ages ago gray-haired grannies bundled their hair into top-knots or chignons; and in this modern day and age, the pat way of dealing with gray hair has been to cut and curl it. But with gray hair, as with any other kind, you should feel free to make your own rules. A smart, modern look for gray hair that I prefer is one that is cut shorter and all one length. A layered look tends to make the face look older, and I would advise avoiding it if you have a great deal of gray.

Certainly going gray is not the end of lovely looking hair. If you understand yourself and your hair's possibilities, you'll realize that gray hair can be the beginning of something very beautiful.

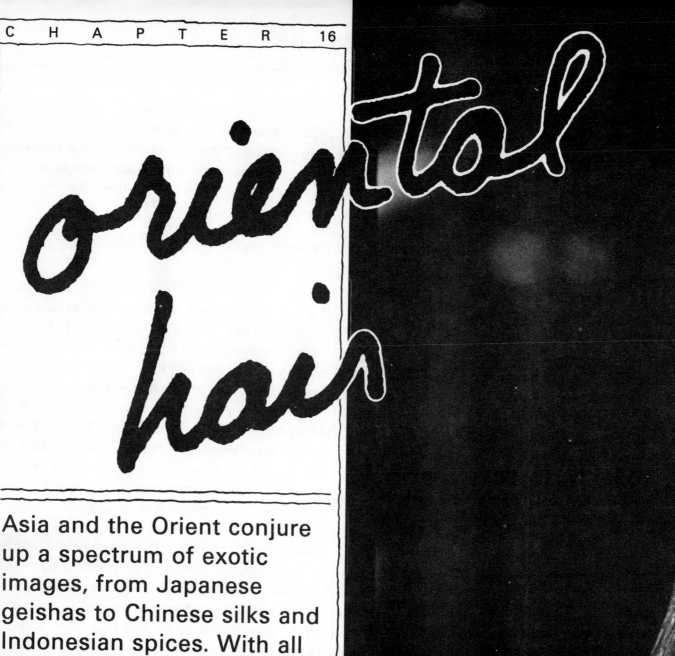

oriental hair

Asia and the Orient conjure up a spectrum of exotic images, from Japanese geishas to Chinese silks and Indonesian spices. With all the differences these many countries and cultures present, there is one aspect common to all their people. And that is the unmistakable beauty of their hair. Strikingly lustrous, usually jet black, almost always arrow-straight, and as shiny as the reflections of sunlight on water.

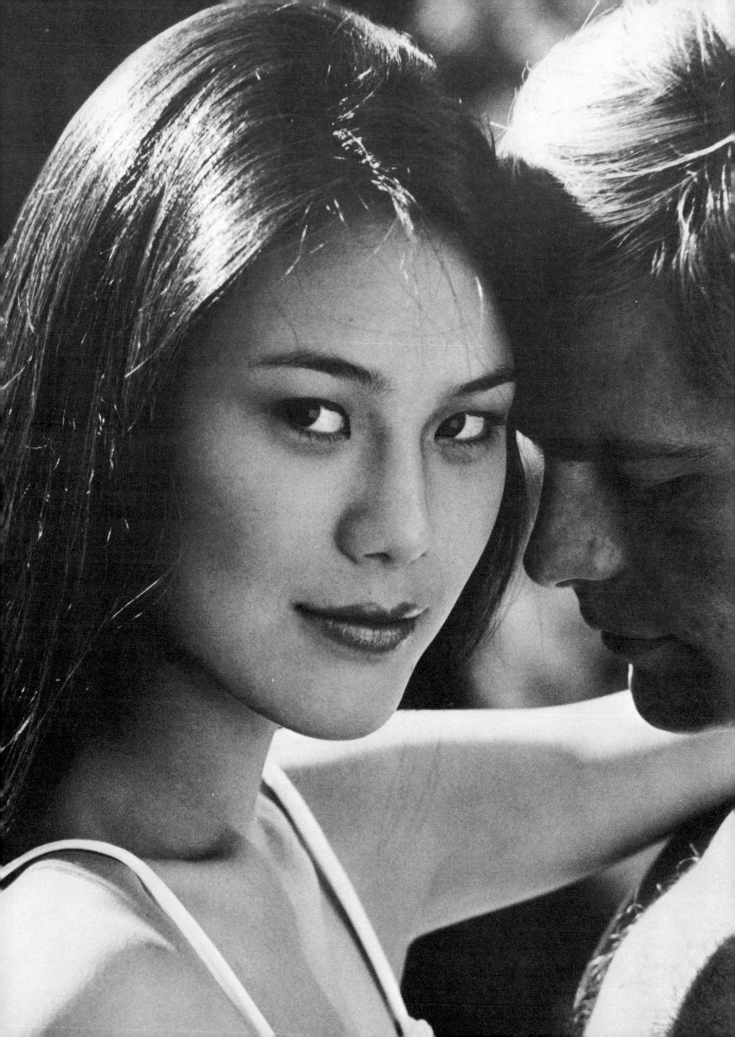

But as beautiful and healthy as it is, Oriental hair is also the most confusing hair to cut and style. And unless a stylist really understands its nature and unique characteristics, the outcome can be less than a happy one. Oriental hair needs special attention, and that's why I've devoted a whole chapter to it.

To begin with, Oriental hair is physiologically different. If you were to view a strand through a microscope you would see that it is rounder than Caucasian and Black hair. In fact, it is the widest in diameter of all hair types. It is characteristically high on both elasticity and tensile strength. These qualities give it exceptional drama, but also a stubborn streak that will try your patience because it will usually do what *it* wants and not what *you* want. But ways have been found handle it.

THE CUT IS THE KEY

Since Oriental hair is very slippery and hard to control, finding a stylist with special skills should be a prime consideration. The stylist must be capable of precise and concentrated cutting, or the results will be disastrous. The stylist should also be aware that the texture of Oriental hair causes a special "spring-back" phenomenon to take place when the hair is cut—its high elasticity causes it to spring or snap back like a rubber band, and it will look much shorter when it's dry. It's important, therefore, to be sure to cut the hair when wet and leave it a bit longer to compensate for its natural springiness. It should be checked again when dry.

The Best Length and Cut. Straight Oriental hair looks and works best chin to shoulder length. If you want to wear your hair naturally straight, my advice is to have it cut all the same length. It can be cut blunt if the hair texture is not too thick. If it is thick, it should be slightly angled at the bottom to eliminate that squared-off "broom" effect, unless that's the effect you're after.

When it comes to length, I always prefer Oriental hair to be on the longer side because it is typically plagued by many cowlicks, and the weight of longer hair helps control this annoying characteristic. A short layered cut on straight hair accentuates this problem, making the hair stand up on end like broom bristles. To avoid this, leave the nape and crown longer.

Naturally wavy hair (an exception among Asians, by the way) should be kept on the short side for easier handling. And if you plan on having a permanent wave or a body wave, keep the hair fairly long; otherwise the resulting length might turn out to be much too short.

Straight Oriental hair can also be cut my "wash-and-wear" way if it has enough of its own bounce. Either let it dry by itself or towel- or finger-dry it (see Chapter 10). However, if the hair is limp and so heavy that its own weight pulls down the bounce, there are ways to add uplift.

How to Add Bounce. Putting some bounce and curl into Asian hair takes an extra measure of patience and skill and, above all, understanding of what you're dealing with.

Blow-drying. When hair is arrow-straight, frequent blow-drying might be necessary to add bounce. This probably will get you a soft curl, but it won't do very much for the health of your hair. So be sure to condition regularly.

Rollers. If you prefer using rollers to set your hair, always use the largest size that will fit into your hand. But don't leave them in until your hair is completely dry. It's better to remove them when your hair is slightly damp—you'll have an easier time creating the look you want.

If you insist on electric rollers, wet the hair slightly first and use end papers before rolling up. This will help prevent frizziness and some of the dryness this harsh electric appliance causes.

Body waves. If you really don't like your straight hair and want more body and movement, try a body wave. It's best on long hair cut all the same length or angled, and also on a layered cut. You'll find that a body wave will be less trouble than constant blow-drying or roller setting.

Perms. When applying a permanent wave to Oriental hair, the timing is extremely important, more important than on any other hair type. Just a few minutes can make the difference between wave and frizz. Also, the rods used should be larger in size than average, and fewer rods should be used overall. I recommend extreme caution when having a permanent wave; if you are considering one, by all means have a professional do it rather than attempting a do-it-yourself home procedure.

Bangs. Bangs are almost synonymous with an "Oriental" look. Maybe they look best on Asian women because their hair seems thicker, straighter, glossier—creating full, shiny bangs, not skimpy wisps. Bangs are more than a great look, too: They keep the hair off the face, and they are masterful cover-ups for any hairline imperfections.

The Oriental influence of bangs inspired my **China Chop**—a cut and look that accentuates the hair's beauty simply because it **is** so simple. Straight or wavy hair can benefit from the strikingly clean lines of the China Chop.

COLOR

Most Oriental hair is black—in some rare cases dark brown—with beautiful shine and great strength. My advice would be not to color it artificially unless you have a graying problem. How can you improve the already naturally beautiful color this hair has? However, if you *really* want to try a different color, use a semipermanent one in the same shade as your own natural shade. Certain elements in the chemicals of perms, or

even excessive exposure to the sun, can give Oriental hair a reddish cast. If this bothers you, I suggest using a semipermanent color one shade lighter than your natural color. But do this only once or twice a year. The less the better, in my book (see Chapter 12).

Gray Hair. Gray hair among Asians usually appears much later in life than it does among Westerners. If it shows up earlier, try a semipermanent color. I don't recommend using a color tint because it is not necessary unless you have over 30 percent gray. If you stick to a semipermanent color, you will spend less time on upkeep and it will not stop you from having a body wave, if that's what you want. Using a color tint on your hair and a permanent wave together will bring out a lot of red and will also dry your hair. So take special care when it comes to chemical process interaction.

CARE AND FEEDING

Because Oriental hair is characteristically straight, it has a tendency to be oily. Straight hair grows flat from the head, allowing the oil from the scalp to travel down the hair shaft more easily. Daily shampooing is a must, along with regular conditioning. But remember, if your hair is oily, applying conditioner only to the ends is the best way to help your hair. Heavy conditioners or heavy-handed applications might only give you the "greasies." And if your hair is chemically treated, a deep treatment from time to time will counteract some of the dryness these processes create.

If your hair gets the best of you every now and then . . . if you long for curls or blonde streaks . . . stop for a minute and consider the exceptional beauty of what you've got. Your black, mirror-shiny hair is unique and uniquely yours . . . part of a natural beauty millions of women envy and admire as much as I do.

problems

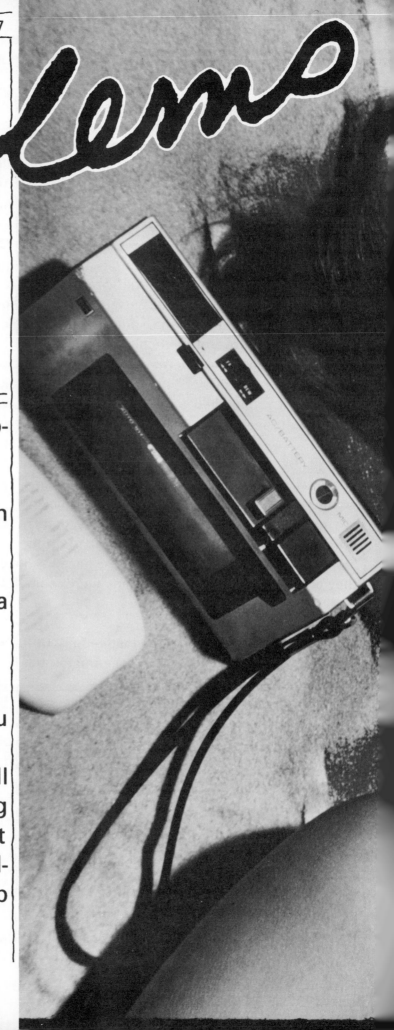

Behind some of the most innocent disguises lurk some of your hair's worst enemies. Who would think that a stylish hat could lead to scalp and hair problems? Who would imagine that the coziness of a well-heated apartment or home could cause dry, dull hair? Certainly no one would ever criticize all those laps you swim to keep trim. But does anyone ever question what all that chlorinated water is doing to your hair? And what about those blow-dryers, rollers, styling combs? Did you ever stop to think that you're "killing" your hair with convenience?

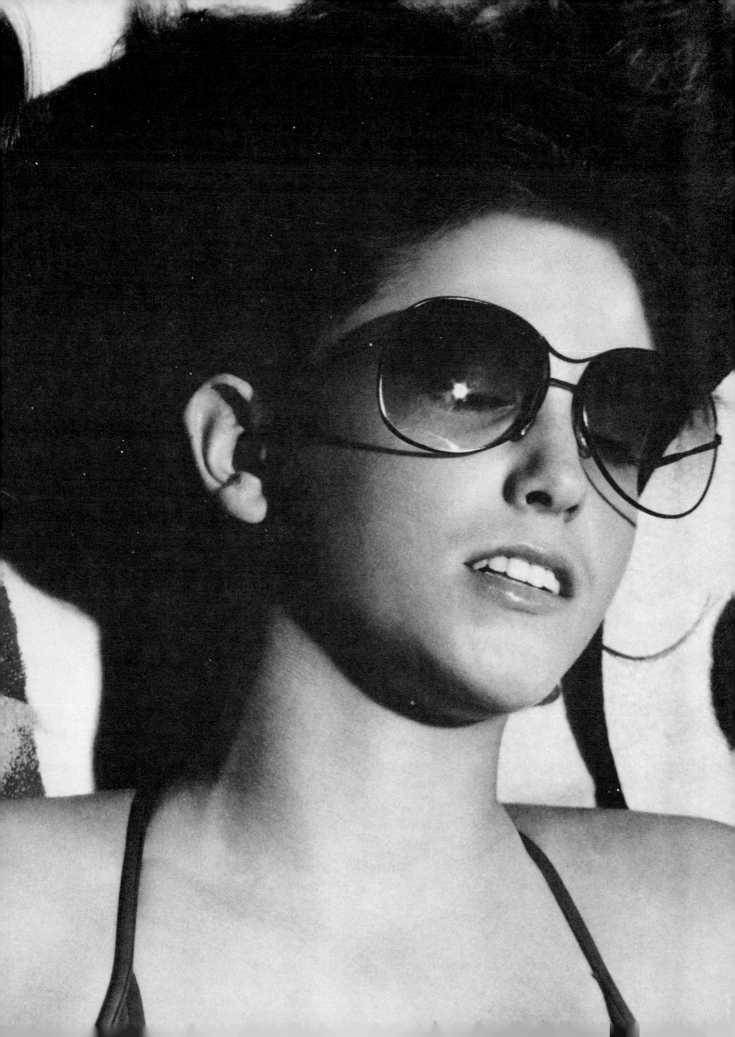

Hair problems come in so many camouflages that it really is difficult to remain aware of and alert to them all. Unfortunately, many women are too slow to recognize a potential hot spot and only do something after the problem is full-blown. The advice I am about to give you stresses the timeless adage that says "an ounce of prevention is worth a pound of cure." Let this be your guiding motto, especially when it comes to having and keeping great-looking hair. Though hair may be tough and tolerate a great deal of abuse, it does have its breaking point. So it's up to you to keep a keen eye on its care and feeding. After all, your hair lives the life *you* lead. It has no other choice.

I have compiled a list of hair problems and hair enemies, along with possible solutions and definite preferences. It is meant for you to use as a handy reference guide when in doubt. And though it might not answer all your questions or attack all the trouble spots, it does cover a fairly broad spectrum of some of the more common hair problems facing the contemporary woman.

EQUIPMENT ENEMIES

We are creatures of convenience, and what seems like a shortcut or quick solution appeals to most of us. This is especially true when it comes to hair equipment—rollers, pins, brushes, electrics, etc. But beware. They do cause considerable damage.

Enemies		*Preference*
Rubber bands. These pull and stretch the hair and cause breakage.	1.	Coated rubber bands, ribbon or yarn, plastic clips, pipe cleaner-type ornaments, plastic ponytail rings.
Metal barrettes. They have sharp metallic edges that break hair.	2.	Barrettes with rubber locks, comb ornaments.
Metal hair clips. They also have sharp edges that break hair.	3.	Plastic clips or coated bobby pins.
Brush rollers. The brushes split and break hair.	4.	Rollers without brushes or plastic rollers. They won't break or pull hair.
Mesh brush rollers for sleeping. They pull hair when you rest on them and also hurt the scalp and so are uncomfortable.	5.	Sponge rollers are better, softer, and won't pull hair.
Brushes with metal bristles. They pull, break, and split hair.	6.	Nylon, natural, or a mix of natural-nylon bristle—all are more gentle and prevent hair breakage.
Metal combs with any size teeth. They're too harsh and tend to break the hair.	7.	Rubber or plastic combs, but only those with large, widely spaced teeth. Small, fine teeth break hair and should never be used.
Metal hair pics. Their sharp teeth are harsh and cause hair breakage.	8.	Hard rubber or nylon pics with widely spaced teeth eliminate hair breakage.
Wrong choice of brush for preshampoo, postshampoo, or regular brushing. The wrong brush will pull hair unnecessarily and break it.	9.	Select the appropriate brush for the appropriate task. There are differences in bristle, shape, firmness (see Chapter 7).

| Excessive blow-drying. It dries out hair, and the pulling action of the brush causes the scorched hair to break. | 10. | Choose the right blow-dryer for your type and texture hair (see Chapter 10). Be sure that the heat wattage is correct for you. Always remove excess water first. When hair is damp, use blow-dryer no closer than 6" from scalp. |

Electric rollers.
They may be practical and speedy, but they are extremely damaging to hair. The high heat dries out hair and causes breakage.

Curling irons 12. Never!

Hair spray 13. Never!

11. If you must, use them with end papers.

Bonnet dryer. 14. Be very careful
Staying under this type of dryer too long will dry out hair. Also, drying too often, even at low heat, will cause a certain amount of hair and scalp dryness.

about drying time. Suggested approximate dryings times: 20/30 minutes for short to medium long hair; 35/45 minutes for long hair.

Hairpieces and wigs. 15. Attach with extreme care,
Because of their weight, they cause hair breakage where they are attached to the hair. Constant use will cut down air circulation and will make hair look dull and lifeless.

especially in the front where the hair is weakest. Be sure to give hair a day off between wearings—let it breathe. Shampoo and condition regularly, even if you feel your hair will be covered so that it "doesn't matter what it looks like."

Hats. 16. Scalps need the circulation
Covered scalps produce increased amounts of oil and perspiration.

of fresh air. If you wear hats a lot, shampoo a lot.

NATURAL ENEMIES

Our growing love for sports, the outdoors, sunshine, and snowtime has also created its own growing list of hair killers. If you swim, sauna, or are part of the fitness generation, here are some enemies to guard against . . . and ways to protect your overall health, including that of your hair.

Enemies *Antidotes*

Chlorinated pool water. 1. Shampoo hair
Can cause bleached blonde hair to turn green—especially if hair is overbleached and exceptionally porous.

as soon as you leave pool and be sure to apply a conditioner.

Sauna. 2. Try applying a cream
Intense high heat causes hair and scalp to become very dry.

conditioner to hair while you're relaxing in the sauna—or, for a special treat, give yourself a deep conditioning like my Double O at the same time.

Sun and salt water.
Overexposure to the sun, especially when combined with exposure to salt water, will result in dry hair and scalp.

Winter "limp."
The biggest sause of limp, flat hair is wearing hats, caps, and hoods—all of which have a tendency to flatten down hair.

Overheated homes.
Moistureless air in homes and apartments and even where you work cause dry hair, skin, and scalp.

Wind.
Causes severe tangling of hair.

3. Wear a sun hat
at the beach or apply conditioner to hair and let the sun activate the conditioning process. Wash hair immediately after leaving the beach.

4. For more fluff
during the cold winter months, try shampooing more often. Also, shake your head when you take off your hat. This will aerate and fluff up your hair.

5. Supplement daily
with conditioner and periodic deep treatments. A humidifier will also help.

6. Try wearing a scarf or hat, or
keep hair gathered in a ponytail or braid.

TREATMENT ENEMIES

We're always doing something to our hair, whether it's brushing it, shampooing it, cutting it. But take care. These daily and seemingly innocent treatments can cause lots of hair damage—especially if done incorrectly. Here are some proper ways and methods to help keep your hair healthy.

Enemies

Every-which-way motion while shampooing. This gets your hair all tangled when it's wet—its most vulnerable time—and almost guarantees breakage.

Pulling hair while trying to detangle it after shampooing.
This causes it to snap like a broken elastic.

Razor cuts.
They leave thin ends, which are vulnerable to more splitting.

Singeing split ends.
This damages hair and makes split ends even more noticeable.

Teasing.
It causes severe hair breakage and split ends. It also creates a very old-fashioned look.

Helps

1. Work shampoo in, following the length of the hair.
Use a gentle motion to reduce knots and hair breakage. Remember, wet hair is weak hair (see Chapter 8).

2. *Never* pull hair in attempting to detangle it. Use the correct technique and tools (see Chapters 7 and 8). Also use the right conditioner; this will help reduce the problem of tangled hair.

3. Use scissors to cut hair.

4. Snip tips of hair with scissors.

5. For added volume, try simply bending over and brushing your hair away from your head. Then flip it back and you'll have instant fullness.

Pomade.
It picks up dust—and your hair is not furniture!

Excessive bleaching, coloring, permanent waving, straightening. Any excessive use of chemicals will damage the hair structure, causing hair to look dull, drab, and even to break.

6. Try another way to add shine to your hair, such as one of my natural conditioning treatments in Chapter 9.

7. Avoid back-to-back chemical processing. Wait an appropriate time in between to give your hair a restoring period.

"JUST-BECAUSE" ENEMIES

It's not always a matter of "things" causing problems with hair. Sometimes it's just because our hair or scalp or even our life-styles create damaging or hard-to-manage conditions. You may be dieting, or under medication, or tense from a new job. Or you just may have been born with frizzy or curly hair that you think you can't do anything with. But you *can* do something about all these problems.

Enemies

Dry hair.
Damaged hair tends to look dry, especially if some of the natural oils are depleted.

Oily hair.
Hair that becomes oily six hours after shampooing, especially the first 2" from the roots, indicates an oily scalp. Oiliness shows up more when hair is short, fine, and close to the scalp; when you do not shampoo enough; or when you use too much of the wrong conditioner.

Dull hair.
When hair cuticles are damaged, they do not lie flat, and therefore can't reflect light and shine. Roughing up of the cuticle can be caused by excessive use of chemicals, teasing, hair sprays, setting lotions, wigs, hairpieces, hats, improper diet, poor circulation to scalp, stress, and certain medications. It can also be caused by using the wrong shampoo (some dandruff shampoos, for example, can be very harsh), not shampooing enough, or not conditioning after shampooing.

Solutions

1. Try less frequent colorings, perms, other chemical treatments. Switch to low-heat blow-drying or none at all for a while. Apply conditioner daily. Try a deep oil-wrap treatment (see Chapter 9).

2. The best remedy is frequent shampooing. And when you condition, apply the conditioner only to the ends of the hair.

3. Try to evaluate the source of your problem by a series of tests. If you are doing any of the listed "no's," stop for a while and see if there is an improvement in your "shine level."

Oily scalp.
This condition is caused by a high level of hormones that control the production of the sebaceous (oil) glands.

Dry scalp.
This condition is caused by improper diet; by not rinsing hair thoroughly; using beer as a setting lotion; cold weather; overheated rooms; too much blow-drying.

Dandruff.
Dandruff usually occurs on an oily scalp when the cells of the scalp age, dry, and fall off in flakes.

Perspiration.
The waste materials in perspiration include some salts. Salt dries the hair and its gritty residue causes tangles and breakage.
Diet pills, birth control pills.
Both can cause shifts in the hormonal balance, which in turn affects hair.

High fever.
Can cause a certain amount of hair fall-out if prolonged and severe, because it will result in a nitrogen loss.
Stress and tension.
Both increase the production of oil to the scalp, causing the greasies and dandruff. It is also thought that stress creates a tightening effect on the capillaries that feed the hair follicles. This in turn cuts down on the amount of oxygen and nutrients reaching the hair and can cause the hair to fall out.

4. After puberty, hormone production usually levels off, but the scalp can continue to be oily for several more years. When shampooing, use only one soaping. The more you shampoo, the more you massage the scalp—and the more it will tend to secrete oil.

5. Check your scalp at least once a week to determine its condition. Gently scrape your fingernail over the scalp. If a white, grainy deposit appears, it is a telltale sign of dry scalp. If unchecked it can lead to severe problems, such as scabs, dandruff, or psoriasis.

6. Normally, regular shampooing and brushing remove the flakes.
If not, try a special dandruff-fighting shampoo until the condition clears up. Dandruff that is accompanied by redness or broken skin might indicate psoriasis or seborrheic dermatitis. Check with your doc-tor before attempting to treat the problem.

7. If you engage in sports that cause you to perspire heavily, it is best to shampoo your hair right after finishing the activity so that your hair will look as great as your body feels.

8. Rapid weight loss can cause hair loss. Birth control pills often lead to increased hair growth (because they stimulate higher estrogen levels)—but sometimes they can have quite the opposite effect. Pay attention to hair nutrition whenever you're taking pills that will alter your body's chemistry.

9. If you have had a high fever, make sure you're now getting enough vitamins. When the body is nutritionally impoverished, there is less hair growth.

10. Try shampooing daily with a mild shampoo. Also, try relaxing during stressful times; yoga, exercise, dance class, meditation—all do wonders in taking the mind to pleasant places.

Hair fall-out. 11. This is still one of the great unsolved mysteries, but certain causes have been linked to hair loss, such as toxic amounts of vitamin A; postpartum alopecia (hair loss after pregnancy, due to a shift in the hormonal balance); chemotherapy; stress and tension; certain hormone-altering drugs; thyroid imbalance; anemia; high fever; diabetes.

Broken hairline. 12. When all of the causes mentioned are corrected, most hair will grow back. So don't panic. And in the meantime, you can compensate by trying some of the looks in Chapter 6.

Very common problem, caused by incorrect brushing technique or using the wrong brush; too much pulling and too much heat when you blow-dry; sleeping with rollers; keeping hair too tightly pulled back from face; medications that affect hair loss, including birth control pills; stress and tension; overprocessing with chemicals.

Frizzy hair. 13. Work with frizzy hair, not against it. It does not have to be unruly or shapeless. A great cut makes all the difference in the world. Curly hair can look good short or long, but frizzy hair looks better and is more manageable when short. Left natural, it will dry in a perfectly shaped halo. As a change, it's easy to blow frizzy hair straight for a smoother look. If you want your long frizzy hair straight, the best result comes from first setting the hair and blow-drying it afterward. Frizzy hair, because it tends to be dry, should be conditioned often.

Frizzy hair can look unruly, can be difficult to style—sometimes you can't even get a comb through it—and most of all has a tendency to be dry.

Curly hair in humid weather. 14. Let your hair do what it wants. Stay away from greasy lanolin conditioners. Find one that builds body and shine. Applying straightener will either make your hair arrow-straight so it won't do a thing (then you'll really miss your curl), or it will dry it out so much that it becomes frizzy.

Now that you know what to look for, most every potential hair problem can be headed off at the pass. That's what I call prevention. But knowing is not enough. Application is the other important half of the success formula. Doing what's right is essential to having and keeping more beautiful, healthy hair. The kind you want. And the kind I care about.